Anywhere, Anytime, Any Body Yoga

What Readers Are Saying…

"Emily is a gifted teacher who leads her class to experience what yoga has in store for them that day. Whether the emphasis is on stretching, balance, muscle toning, or restoration, the session is individualized to meet the needs of the student. As she brings each class to a relaxing summation with "eyes closed, nowhere to go, nothing to do," we feel gratitude for her kindness and gentle coaching. Namasté, Emily!"

— Dr. Jo Turner
Naturopathic Physician

"I have been taking yoga from Emily for several years. Emily's love for and joy from teaching her students are present in every one of her sessions. She is passionate about yoga, and compassionate about people! This book is a perfect example—it grew from her desire to show how yoga is able to improve the quality of life for those with physical limitations. She is a wonderful instructor and, more importantly, a person full of loving spirituality."

— Sandy Eto
U.S. Bureau of Reclamation

"I first met Emily when she attended my Yoga classes for the City of Glendale. Several years later she impressed me by going for Certification as a teacher herself, her special training being in Geriatric Yoga. She taught a Chair Yoga class for the Sun Health organization and became the most popular teacher they had."

— Reverend Ted Czukor

DEDICATION

*This book is dedicated
to all of my yoga students
who constantly prod and inspire me.*

Ordering

Trade bookstores in the U.S. and Canada please contact:

Publishers Group West
1700 Fourth Street, Berkeley CA 94710
Phone: (800) 788-3123   Fax: (800) 351-5073

Hunter House books are available at bulk discounts for textbook course adoptions;
to qualifying community, health-care, and government organizations;
and for special promotions and fund-raising.
For details please contact:

Special Sales Department
Hunter House Inc., PO Box 2914, Alameda CA 94501-0914
Phone: (510) 865-5282   Fax: (510) 865-4295
E-mail: ordering@hunterhouse.com

Individuals can order our books from most bookstores,
by calling **(800) 266-5592**, or from our website at
www.hunterhouse.com

Anywhere, Anytime, Any Body Yoga

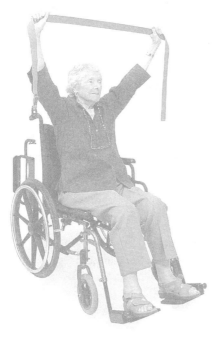

A PRACTICAL GUIDE TO USING YOGA IN EVERYDAY LIFE

Emily Slonina

Hunter House
PUBLISHERS

Hunter House Inc., Publishers
PO Box 2914
Alameda CA 94501-0914

Library of Congress Cataloging-in-Publication Data
Slonina, Emily.
Anywhere, anytime, any body yoga : a practical guide to using yoga in everyday life / Emily Slonina.
p.   cm.
ISBN 978-0-89793-519-7
1. Yoga.   I. Title.
B132.Y6S575 2009
613.7'046—dc22   2009032697

Project Credits

Cover Design	Amy Hagelin
Interior Photographer	Jim Petersen of Sun Camera, Sun City, AZ
Book Design & Production	John McKercher
Copy Editor	Amy Bauman
Proofreader	John David Marion
Editor	Alexandra Mummery
Senior Marketing Associate	Reina Santana
Publicity Coordinator	Sean Harvey
Rights Coordinator	Candace Groskreutz
Customer Service Manager	Christina Sverdrup
Order Fulfillment	Washul Lakdhon
Administrator	Theresa Nelson
Computer Support	Peter Eichelberger
Publisher	Kiran S. Rana

Printed and bound by Bang Printing, Brainerd, Minnesota

Manufactured in the United States of America

9 8 7 6 5 4 3 2 1   First Edition   10 11 12 13 14

Contents

> The numbers beside the illustrations are matched
> to the numbers in the text. When the illustration is
> of a variation of the pose, it is marked Var.

Acknowledgments

My gratitude to all the people who have encouraged and supported my efforts to bring this book to fruition. Also to Laura, who set my vision into motion, and Ed, who refused to let the vision fade.

My heartfelt thanks to Matthew for providing his expertise and services in the preparation of the photographs for print. And a very special thanks goes to all of our models for their endless patience and enthusiasm.

And, finally, I thank all of my teachers and all of the teachers before me for passing the yoga tradition on. The divine light in me honors the divine light in you.

Namasté,

Emily

Important Note

The material in this book is intended to provide a review of information regarding the practice of yoga. Every effort has been made to provide accurate and dependable information and the contents of this book have been compiled through professional research and in consultation with medical professionals. However, much of yoga is physical movement. Although it gives us an opportunity for relaxation, stress re-education, and relief from aches and pains, the risk of injury is always present. Before undertaking a new exercise regimen or doing any of the exercises or suggestions contained in this book, it is recommended that you consult your health-care professional. For example, individuals who suffer from high blood pressure or those with knee or hip replacements may find some poses not appropriate. Although yoga is helpful, it is never intended as a substitute for medical attention.

The author, publisher, editors, and professionals quoted in the book cannot be held responsible for any error, omission, or dated material in the book. The author and publisher are not liable for any damage or injury or other adverse outcome of applying the information in this book in an exercise program carried out independently or under the care of a licensed trainer or practitioner. If you have questions concerning the application of the information described in this book, consult a qualified and trained professional.

From Our Models

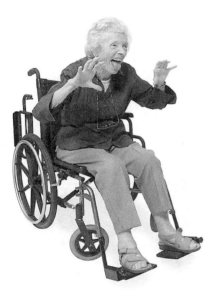

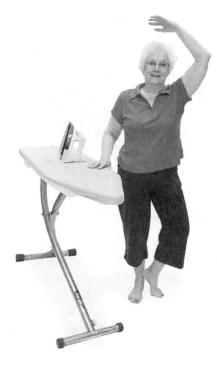

Marlene: "I've missed only two months of classes in the last four years, and that was when I had a full knee replacement in 2008. I know positively that the yoga helped speed my recovery."

Jean: "I started practicing yoga on the advice of my doctor. I find it helps with pain relief and helps keep my muscles strong. It allows me to function better."

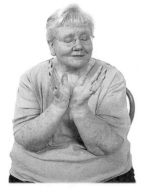

Shirley: "Amazing things happen when I breathe deeply, go inside myself, and use calming imagery. To become relaxed, serene, and accepting is wonderful — and my blood pressure can drop 25 points. Yoga classes have been life changing for me. Yay for yoga!"

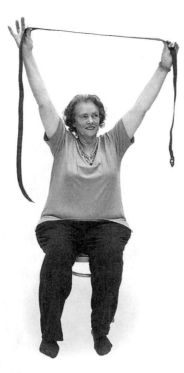

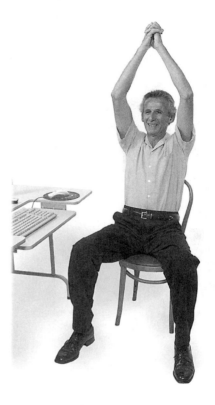

Rosemary: "The Sciatic Stretch has relieved the pressure on that nerve and has eased the pain and numbness in my legs and feet. While traveling in a plane recently, I found enough room while seated to do some yoga stretches — pain gone!"

Ed: "I have lower-back and shoulder problems. The yoga stretching relieves the muscular tension and allows me to continue to work. I'm new to yoga, and I can't believe how something that looks so simple can help so much."

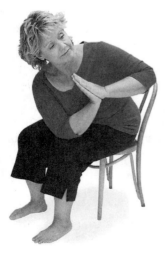

Carlyn: "It's hard to condense my feelings — yoga has helped me live more peacefully. It nourishes my body and mind. I feel more fluid. I crave its movement and plan to practice it the rest of my life."

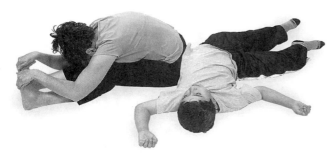

Hildelenia (and Alex): "I love practicing yoga with my grandkids as a fun way of strengthening our relationship and encouraging a healthy practice for self esteem and awareness, mental focus, stress relief, and a strong body."

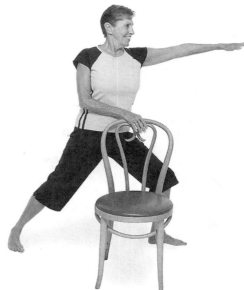

Bebe: "I just love it! When I started in class, I could hardly bend into any of the poses. But now I feel so much more limber. It's a wonderful way to get into touch with one's self."

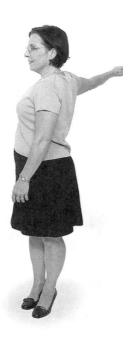

Sharon: "I practice yoga because I have a medical condition that causes muscle and joint pain. Yoga has allowed me to significantly decrease the amount of pain medication I need."

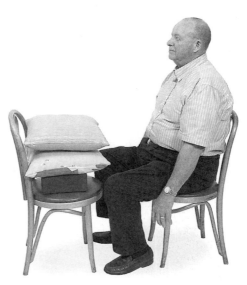

Don: "Very recently I was diagnosed with asthma. I am curious to see how yoga breathing will help with the symptoms."

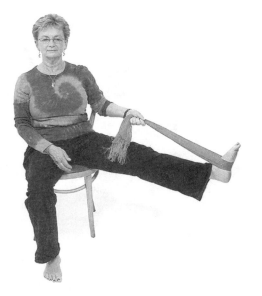

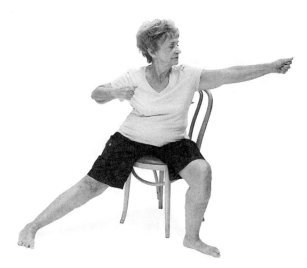

Patty: "I was twenty-three when I started yoga. I am sixty-two now. I learned it from a book. It has brought balance and energy to my life wherever, whenever, and in the midst of whatever. I love it."

Flo: "I practice chair yoga to manage my scoliosis. The poses are not difficult, and they really help. My favorite is the Side-Angle Pose."

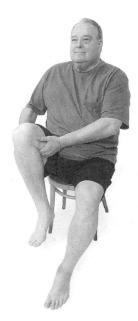

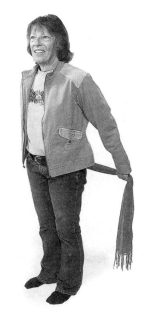

Neil: "After practicing yoga, I feel like I have just received a full body massage."

Sandy: "I love yoga! It is a perfect zero-impact exercise that stretches all my muscles."

Introduction

Traditionally, yoga has been considered a path toward deeper meaning—a union of mind, body, and spirit. Two questions you might ask yourself: How can I begin to use this five-thousand-year-old discipline? And why do I want to? This book will teach you simple yoga principles that you can incorporate into your daily life—while sitting in a chair, lying on a bed, working at the office, traveling, standing in the shower, doing housework. These exercises can be used just about anywhere, anytime, by anybody. And as for the *why*—simply put, because they make you feel good!

When you hear the word *yoga,* what do you picture in your mind? Do you see a lean, muscular man sitting with his legs crossed and his hands resting on his knees? Or do you perhaps see an incredibly flexible woman contorted into a strange position? Both of these images can be correct. Many of us, however, may not have even seen or touched our toes since we were teenagers. Some of us are not able to transition easily from standing to sitting on the floor. Just the thought of standing on our heads may make others of us feel dizzy. Also, in today's society, many of us have very busy schedules and are unable to dedicate much time to perfecting yoga poses. But it is not necessary to plan ahead to practice yoga. A few minutes here and a few minutes there will add up and can make a difference in the quality of our lives. And you can not only do the gentle yoga exercises in this book anywhere and anytime, you can do most of them regardless of the kind of body you have or how fit or flexible you are.

Traditionally, yoga has been practiced to attain knowledge, serenity, and enlightenment. Yoga can also create skeletal realignment, release tension, and modify old mental and emotional patterns. Our minds live in the future, always wondering about what is going to happen next. Our bodies live in the past, holding on to every memory, including the traumas we have experienced. When we practice yoga, our intent is to bring the mind and the body together in the present moment, allowing change to take place.

The benefits of yoga include improving balance, decreasing stress, increasing flexibility, strengthening bones, stabilizing blood pressure, reducing pain and injuries, developing and toning muscles, and helping us age more gracefully. Learning simple breathing techniques aids in calming our chattering minds and helps us focus and de-stress our busy lives.

Our bodies remember movements on a cellular level. When we practice balance, our bodies will recall what to do should we begin to fall or trip. Our muscles have memory and will respond quickly when the need arises. Adding yoga to your life could very well be the start of something much deeper. It may surprise you to find that as you become more flexible in your body, you become more flexible in mind and spirit. By practicing yoga just a few minutes every day, you may see changes occur almost immediately.

Setting an Intention

My intention in writing this book is to show that yoga practice need not be intimidating. For many exercises, you are shown how the classic yoga pose might look. Then, we have photographed people with different needs to show one or more modified poses. Included are additional visuals, which are not always described but are for you to use as inspiration. We deliberately photographed regular, everyday people, not advanced students or masters, and captured them adapting the pose to their body's abilities. Our models vary in age and health condition. Some have arthritis, fibromyalgia, scoliosis, back and/or chronic pain, and heart disease. Rest assured: When done correctly and with awareness, modified poses are just as effective as classical poses. Students of chair yoga experience the same physical, mental, and spiritual benefits as do the students who practice on a mat on the floor. That is the mantra of this book: Yoga can be done anywhere, anytime, and by/with any body.

We encourage you to use your imagination and creativity. When a pose seems too difficult for you, stop, breathe, and ask yourself, "How can I make this pose work for me and my body today?" Each day you may get a different answer. Learn to modify the poses so that each is comfortable and safe for you. I invite you to visualize yourself in a pose before engaging in it. Think of it like rehearsing a play. After all, the intention of yoga is not to see how far you can stretch or bend to touch your toes. Please remain mindful and be aware of what your body is saying to you. **The phrase "no pain; no gain" does not apply to yoga.** Use this book as a guide but always listen to your feelings and sensations. The greatest teacher is within you!

It is my hope that by incorporating even a small measure of yoga into your life, you will feel a profound difference, and you will be inspired to learn more. I encourage you to take a class from a qualified teacher and continue to explore more fully what yoga can offer you.

Namasté.

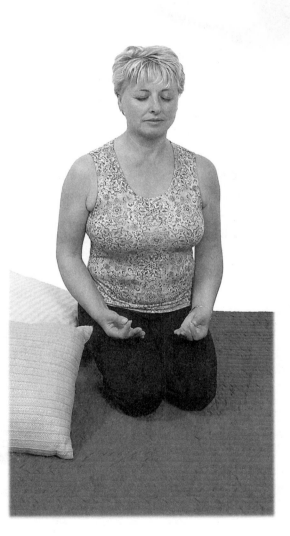

A Few Starting Notes

Before beginning your yoga practice, here are a few things you should know. What you are about to read is referred to throughout the book. Knowing these basics will help you create each pose with ease and bring you greater benefits.

1. Always breathe in and out through your nose unless instructed otherwise. As a yogi, I believe that the nose is for breathing and the mouth is for talking and eating. You are given hints as to when to inhale and when to exhale for most poses. Always continue breathing at your own rhythm and pace. Using your breath is the essence of yoga. When you pay attention to your breathing patterns and intentionally slow your breath, you become more focused and balanced.

2. Many of the poses in the book are done sitting in a chair. It is important to use a straight-back chair without casters or rollers and, preferably, without arms. There is only one pose in the book that requires a chair with arms. And whenever you use a chair, please ensure that it is situated on a nonslip surface. (A sticky yoga mat works very well for this.)

3. Posture and body alignment are important. When the instructions say, "Sit tall in your chair," I mean this: Place both your feet solidly on the ground approximately 4–6 inches apart, and point your toes straight ahead. Your knees should be positioned directly above your ankles. Sit with a straight back, with your shoulders relaxed, away from your ears, and directly above your hips. Your chin is parallel to the floor. Visualize an imaginary string at the crown of your head, gently lifting you up and creating space between each vertebra. If your feet do not touch the floor when you are sitting, place a folded blanket under them. If the chair is too low for you, sit on a folded blanket for elevation.

4. When practicing standing poses, proper foot placement is also important. Your body's weight should be distributed evenly on both feet.

Think of the sole of each foot as having four roots:

- one at the ball of your foot directly under the big toe
- one at the ball of your foot directly under your pinkie toe
- one on each side of your heel

Deliberately root these four points to the earth. Visualize pulling energy up through your feet, ankles, legs, hips, and torso, giving you strength and balance.

During your yoga practice, please remember that a stretch is good, a dull ache is okay, but pain is never acceptable. Also remember that yoga is not a competitive sport. Listen to your body; honor what it is capable of doing today. If you encounter pain, stop or slow down, breathe and try the pose again with less effort and determination. Sometimes it is best to skip a pose entirely. The practice of yoga is a journey, not a destination.

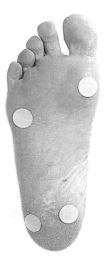

The four roots of the foot

Breathing

Breathing is an involuntary bodily function. Often we are not even aware of it. The purpose of inhaling and exhaling is to bring clean air (oxygen) into the lungs and then to expel the old, stagnant air (carbon dioxide) from the body. Have you ever watched a baby breathe? You will notice that when babies breathe, their bellies, backs, and sides balloon as they inhale. Unfortunately, due to stress, many of us lose that ability at a fairly early age.

Try this: Lightly place one hand on your chest and one on your belly. Breathe normally for a few moments and be aware of the movement of each or your hands. Which hand is moving more than the other? If it is the one resting on your belly, congratulate yourself! If the hand resting on your chest is moving more, then the instruction on the next page will be very useful to you. In the meantime, be aware that you are breathing mostly into your chest, which means you are not taking in enough air to fill your lungs to their capacity. As chest breathers, we must breathe more often and faster, hyperventilating and making our heart work harder than necessary.

The Three-Part Breath, described on the next page, is also known as diaphragmatic breathing. It allows our lungs to fill and empty completely. It maximizes our oxygen intake and aids in expelling carbons. It nourishes our muscles and organs, including our brain. With practice, this should become our standard way of breathing. Practice it anywhere, anytime—on the bus, in the car, standing in line at the grocery store, watching television—and so on.

During your yoga practice, we recommend breathing in and out through your nose, unless otherwise stated. Breathing in the air is filtered, and breathing out the breath is slowed, thus calming your nervous system. Although some breathing techniques used for yoga require breath retention, these will not be addressed in this book.

The Three-Part Breath

Sitting tall or lying comfortably on your back, place one hand on your abdomen and the other on your chest just below your collar bones. Begin by inhaling through your nose. Send the air into your belly, until you feel your hand rise. Then bring the breath toward your rib cage, allowing it to expand. Finally, let your breath rise toward the upper chest, feeling your other hand rise. On the exhale, reverse the process by expelling the air from your chest first, then your rib cage and finally your belly. The breath will become wavelike. Pause when you need to and then repeat. Once you have mastered the process, you will not need to place your hands on your body; your cells will remember how to do this, and this can become your new way of breathing.

Please be aware that beginners may become a bit light-headed or dizzy. If this happens, it is because your brain is not familiar with the extra intake of breath. Do not be alarmed. Stop, breathe normally, and then resume. Practice often—a little bit at a time—until you are accustomed to it.

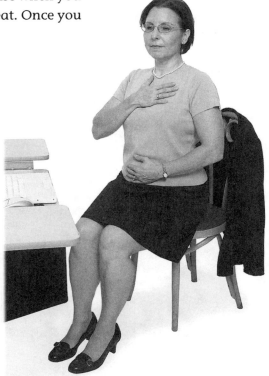

Benefits: Diaphragmatic breathing helps control anxiety, mental and physical stress, and tension. It is beneficial for conditions such as migraines, insomnia, depression, and chronic pain.

Breathing Tip: Another way to think of the diaphragmatic breathing process is to imagine that you are an empty glass. As you would fill an empty glass of water, so you fill your body. First you fill the bottom, then the middle, and finally the top. When you drink, you empty the top first, then the middle, and finally the bottom.

Or imagine an accordion. During the inhale, it expands; the exhale contracts or squeezes the air out.

Be creative. Use a mental image that resonates with you.

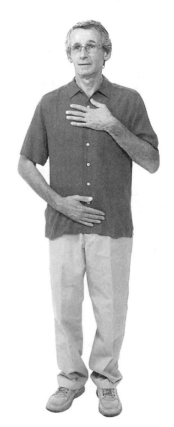

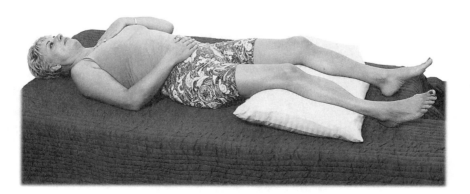

Three Other Breathing Exercises

While the Three-Part Breath is important in our daily lives, there are also times for specialized breathing. The following are three other techniques to try. Each has its own purpose and results.

Alternate-Nostril Breathing

With eyes either focused on the tip of your nose or between your eyebrows, lightly rest your right thumb on your right nostril and your pinkie and ring fingers on your left nostril (1). Your index and middle fingers rest between your eyebrows.

Inhale fully through both nostrils. With your thumb, close your right nostril and breathe out through your left nostril (2). With your right nostril still closed, breathe in through your left nostril. Close your left nostril with your ring and little fingers, release the right nostril, and breathe out (3). This completes one full round.

On your next inhale, breathe in through your right nostril and then breathe out through your left one. Continue, always inhaling thorough the nostril out of which you have just exhaled.

If you are new to breathing techniques, begin with just a few rounds of this practice and increase the number of rounds as you become more comfortable.

1

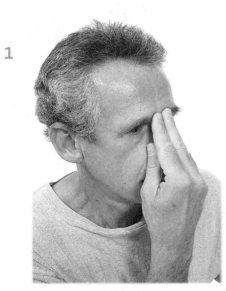

Right view

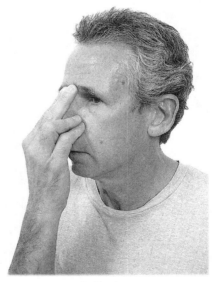

Left view

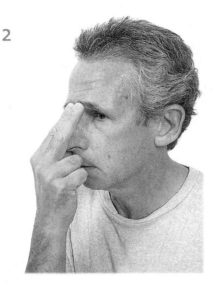

2

If you begin to feel light-headed, this may be because you are receiving more oxygen than what you are used to. If this occurs, simply stop, breathe normally, and then resume later with fewer rounds.

Benefits: Alternate-nostril breathing aids in sinus- and tension-headache relief. Use it to balance your left and right brain hemispheres. This technique is particularly helpful in relieving stress and anxiety. It is also known to reduce cravings.

Travel and Sleep Tip: This form of breathing is effective in reducing travel anxiety. Use it to relax and sleep on a long flight. It also aids in reducing air pres-

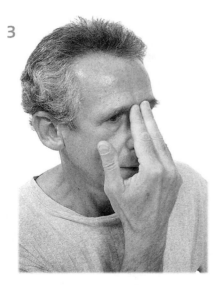

3

Right view

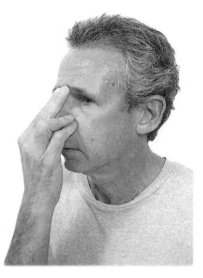

Left view

sure changes during takeoff and landing. You might also try it as a boredom reliever.

The Cooling Breath

With your lips slightly parted, curl the sides of your tongue upward. Take a deep inhale through your mouth and exhale through your nose. You will feel the cooling effects first on your tongue and then throughout your body. Continue breathing this way for several rounds.

Modification: If you are unable to curl your tongue, breathe through your mouth as if you were sipping through a straw. Again, breathe out through your nose.

Benefits: This technique aids in lowering body temperature.

Tip: When you are outside in hot weather, riding in a hot vehicle, or finishing a sweaty workout, try this breath for an immediate drop in body temperature. Ladies: Try this to ease the intensity of your next hot flash.

The Lion's Breath

Sitting tall, inhale through your nose, filling your lungs to their capacity. Exhale through your mouth while raising your hands about shoulder high in front of you (like a lion's paws), spreading your fingers wide, and sticking out your tongue as far as you are able. Imagine your tongue trying to

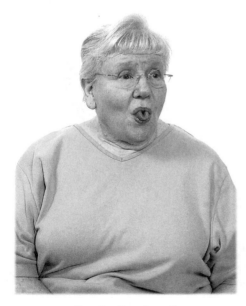

The Cooling Breath

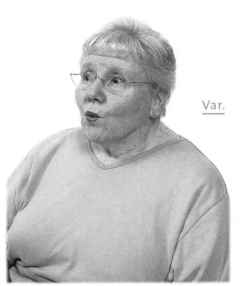

Var.

reach your chin. Your eyes are open or closed and gazing upward. The exhalation is long and slow. Invite your navel to gently move toward your spine, emptying the last bit of remaining breath. Repeat this at least three times.

Benefits: The Lion's Breath is a wonderful stress buster! When gazing upward, it works the optical nerve. It exercises your hands and fingers. And it is a great chest decongestant that also massages the tissues housed in your throat, enhancing your sensory system.

Tip: Laugh at yourself as you practice the Lion's Breath in front of a mirror. It is said that laughter is the best medicine.

During a steamy shower in the morning, Lion's Breath helps break up chest congestion.

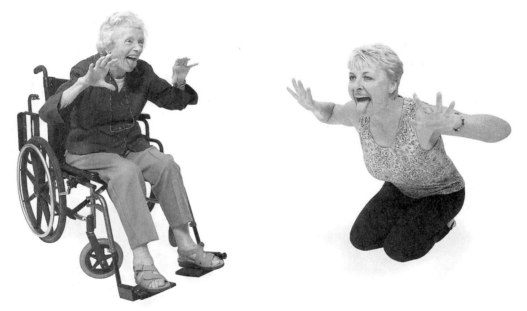

The Lion's Breath

"My husband has heart problems and was sent home from the hospital with a spirometer to measure his breathing. Our son and I witnessed that after practicing the Lion's Breath several times, he could breathe much better, and his skin color quickly returned. We were amazed!" — Ruth

Anytime Neck and Shoulder De-Stressers

Most of us hold a great deal of tension in our neck and shoulders, sometimes due to poor posture, other times due to stress in our lives. The following neck and shoulder de-stressers will help to alleviate some of that tension.

Half-Moon Circles

Sitting tall, take several deep breaths and, on an exhale, allow your chin to drop gently toward your chest (1). Take another deep breath and, again on the exhale, draw an imaginary ¼ circle as you bring your chin toward your right shoulder (2). On another inhale, draw your chin back to your chest (3) and, on the next exhale, draw your chin toward your left shoulder (4). On another inhale, draw your chin back to your chest (5). This completes one round. Repeat as often and as many times as you like. When you are finished, raise your head up slowly and mindfully. Pause. Breathe.

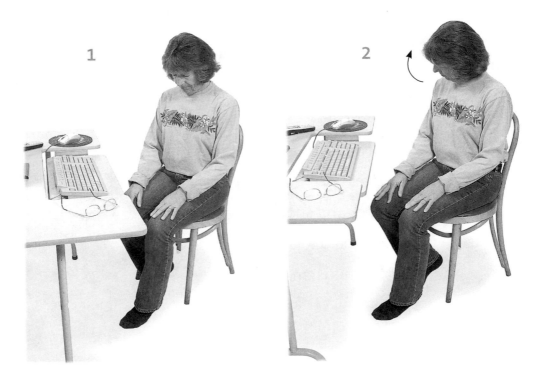

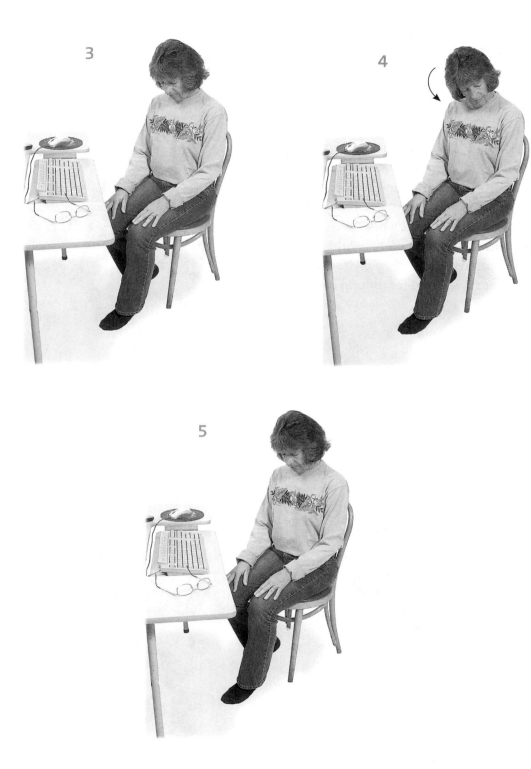

Shoulder Shrugs

Sitting tall (1), inhale deeply through your nose and raise both of your shoulders toward your ears (2). Expel your breath forcefully through your mouth with a big sigh as you deliberately drop your shoulders toward the floor (3). Try not to control or hold on; allow gravity to do its work. Visualize dropping the weight of the world from your shoulders as tension melts away. Repeat as often and for as long as it feels good.

1

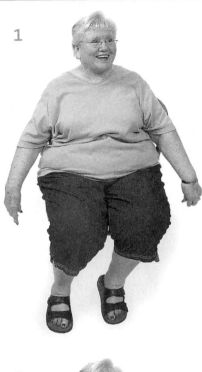

2

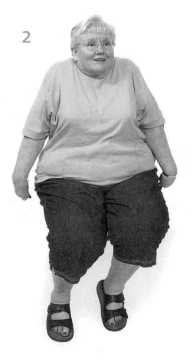

3

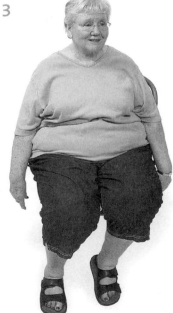

Neck/Shoulder Stretch

Sitting tall (1), take several deep breaths. On an exhale, draw your right ear toward your right shoulder (2). Avoid raising your shoulder to your ear; keep it as relaxed as possible. Breathe deeply and visualize the muscles on the left side of your neck getting longer and more supple. For a deeper stretch, extend your left arm out to the side, as if you were reaching for something (3). And to further deepen the stretch, place your right palm over your left ear or cheek (4). Without pulling, imagine your right elbow getting heavier to increase the elongation of your neck. Continue to

1

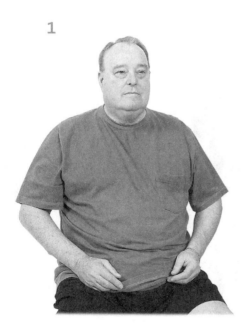

2

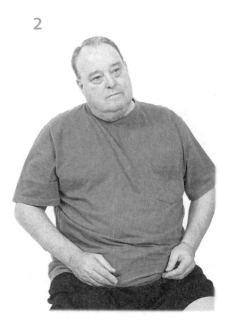

breathe and, when you are finished, mindfully release your right hand, lower your arm, and slowly raise your head. Feel the difference in the dis-tance between your ear and shoulder on your left side compared to that on your right side. Repeat the same on the opposite side.

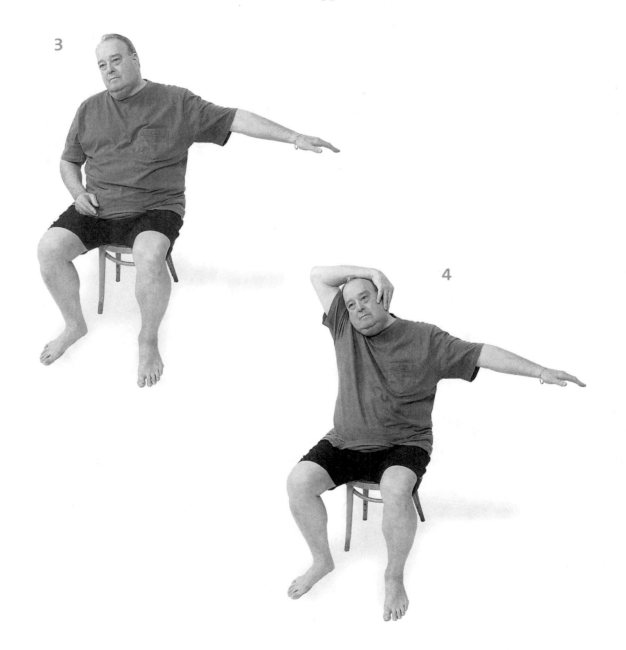

3

4

Shoulder Rolls/Squeezes

Sitting tall (1), on an inhale, shrug your shoulders to your ears (2). On an exhale, squeeze your shoulder blades toward each other as if trying to hold a pencil or coin between them (3). While still squeezing, lower your shoulders toward the floor (4). Repeat as often as you like. Take a moment to notice the energy flowing freely in your upper back and shoulder area.

1

Front view

Back view

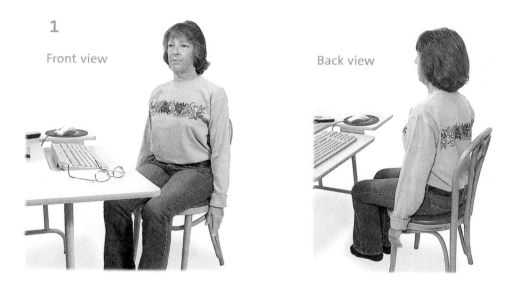

2

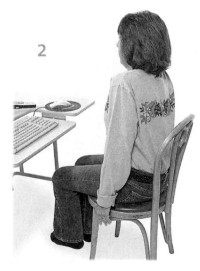

3

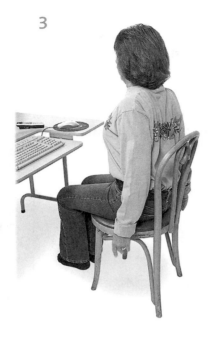
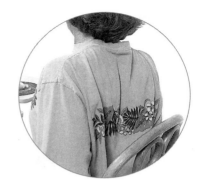

4

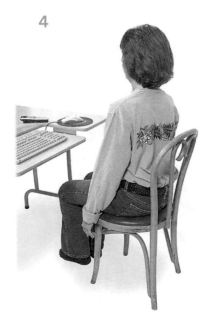

Elbow and Shoulder Circles

Sitting tall, cross your arms and hold both of your elbows at navel height in front of you (1). On an inhale, draw your elbows to the right and then up toward the top of your head (2). On an exhale, complete the circle by bringing your elbows to the left and then down toward the thighs (3). Repeat 3–4 times and then switch the direction of the movement.

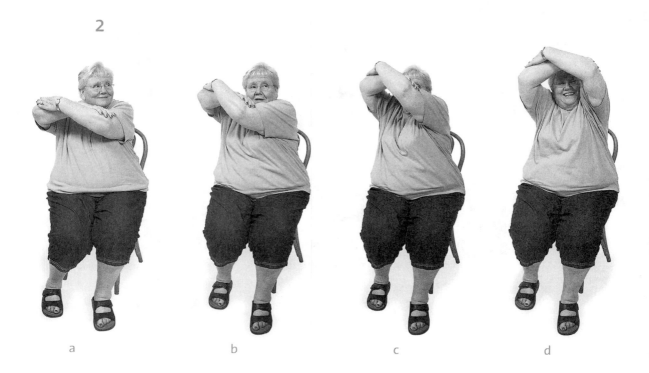

1

2

a

b

c

d

Benefits: Stress easily accumulates in our neck, shoulders, and upper back. Elbow and shoulder circles will encourage blood flow. Often they can relieve headaches and fatigue. Consistent daily practice will slowly increase range of motion.

Office and Travel Tip: These movements are simple and do not require much space. Try them at your desk, in the airport, during a flight, or after your commute.

3

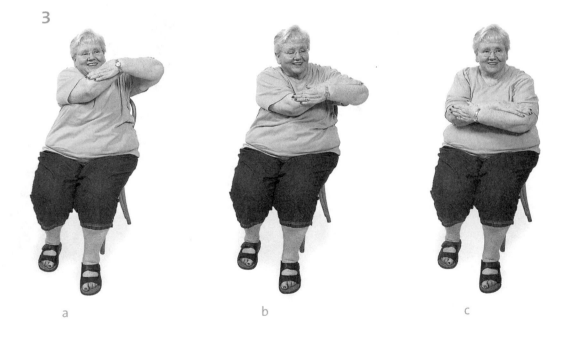

a   b   c

"There was a time when due to rheumatoid arthritis and tendonitis, I could not brush my hair. After six months of chair yoga, I am able to raise my arms. I can drive, clean, and—without pain—comb my hair." — Rhonda

Warm-Ups

It is important to do feet and ankle warm-ups to increase your blood flow before doing any of the standing poses.

Feet and Ankle Warm-Up

Sitting tall in your chair, lift one foot off the floor (1). Slowly and mindfully rotate your ankle several times in one direction and then the other (2). Notice any popping noises or if you feel a difference when you switch the direction of the circles. Next, point and flex your toes several times (3). Notice that when you flex, and your toes are pointing toward the ceiling, the stretch is felt more in the back of your leg. When you point your toes downward, the stretch is felt more prominently in the front of your leg. Repeat the move-ments several times on one foot, and then do the same movements with the other foot.

Benefits: This warm-up strengthens your legs, ankles, and feet and pro-motes increased blood flow.

Tip: Upon rising, and before stepping out of bed in the morning, wake up your lower limbs with these move-ments. Increase circulation with these movements to prevent falls.

1

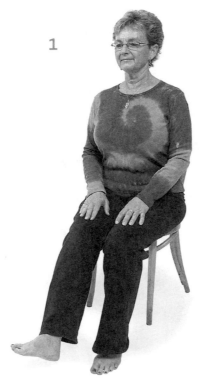

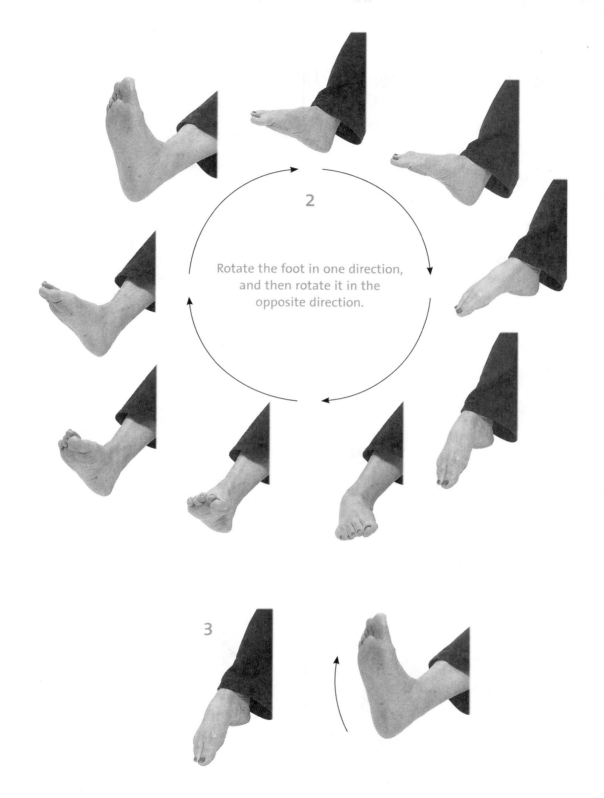

2

Rotate the foot in one direction, and then rotate it in the opposite direction.

3

Yoga for Your Hands and Fingers

Sitting tall in your chair, spread the fingers of your right hand as much as you can until you feel the palm and the webs stretching (1). Relax your shoulders and allow your elbows to feel heavy. Take several deep breaths and, on an exhale, curl your right thumb so it rests inside your palm (2). On each subsequent exhale, mindfully curl the

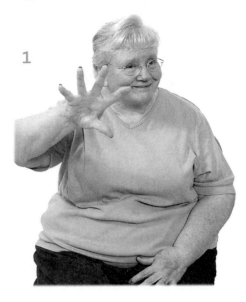

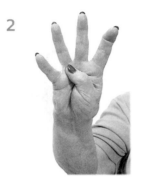

"After much stretching of my arthritic hands, I discovered I can easily reach a full octave on my organ keyboard, something I had not been able to do for years." — Shirley

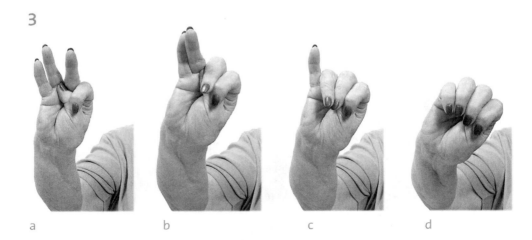

a   b   c   d

rest of your fingers, one at a time, over your thumb (3). On an inhale, extend just your pinkie finger and, on each subsequent inhale, individually extend the rest of your fingers until your palm is spread open again (4). Next, imagine you are squeezing an avocado and close all the fingers at once (5). Slowly release them. Then, wrap your left hand around the thumb of your right hand and massage each knuckle by making small and gentle circles (6).

Softly pull on the fingers to release any trapped air (7). Continue with each finger individually. Now take several breaths and observe the difference in feeling between your hands. Repeat the same sequence with your left hand.

Benefits: The hand and finger exercises ease stiff joints and help alleviate arthritis. They reduce pain and tenderness and increase range of motion.

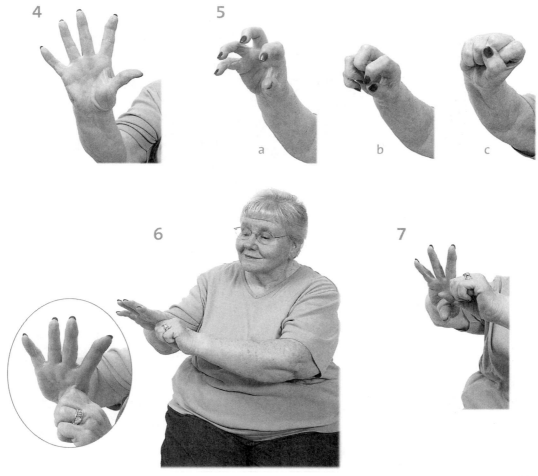

4

5

a

b

c

6

7

Yoga for Your Wrists

Stand facing a desk, table, or other surface. With your palms flat on the surface and fingers facing as much as possible toward you, lean your weight forward for a light stretch, or lean backward for a more intense stretch in the front of your wrists and arms. Hold this stretch for several breaths and then release. Repeat often.

Benefits: The wrist exercises are helpful in relieving carpal tunnel syndrome.

Tip: Any flat surface can be used; depending on the height, the kitchen table or another piece of furniture works well.

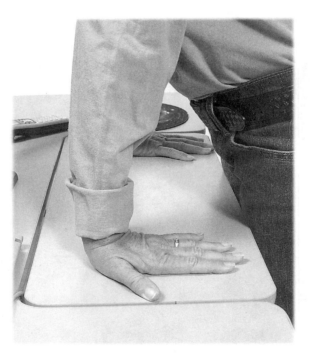

Yoga for Your Eyes

Sit tall in your chair, with your spine and head straight, and bring your right thumb to eye level at arm's length in front of you. While continually gazing at your thumb, and without moving your head, slowly raise your thumb toward the ceiling until it is no longer in your range of focus (1). Then slowly lower your thumb toward the floor (2). Again raise your thumb to eye level and then move your right arm to the right (3). Continue to gaze at your moving thumb without turning your head. Slowly bring the thumb toward you again. Do the same using your left hand and thumb. Repeat several times.

1

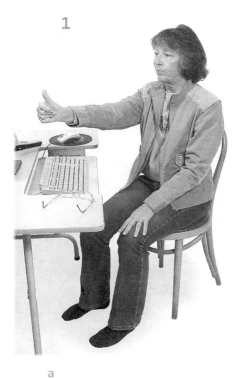

a

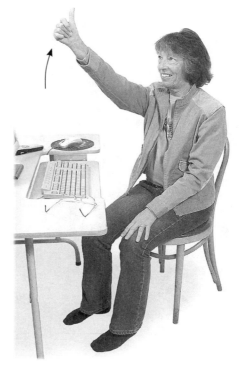

b

To palm your eyes, vigorously rub your hands together to warm them (4). Place your palms over your closed eyes and hold them there as long as you like (5).

Benefits: Yoga exercises for your eyes strengthen your eyes and may improve your vision. These exercises aid in strengthening the muscles that move your eyeball and focus it. They also improve blood flow and alter eye tension.

Office Tip: Take a two-minute break from staring at your computer. Rejuvenate and increase productivity with some yoga for your eyes.

2

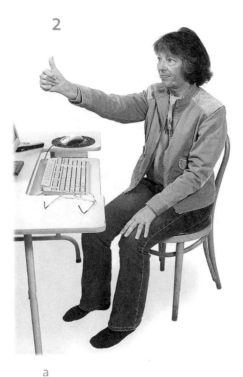

a

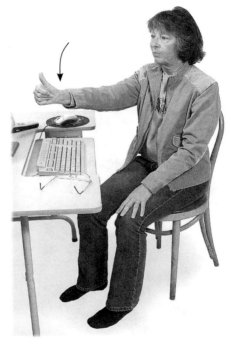

b

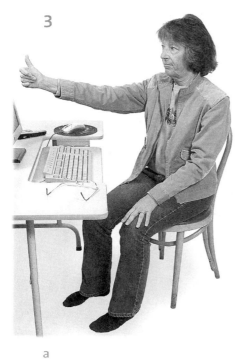

a

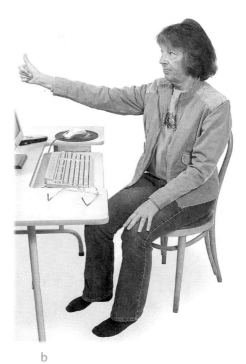

b

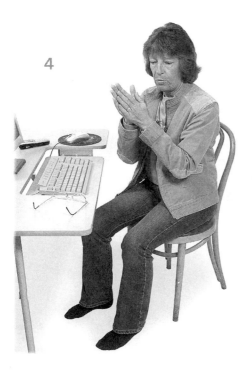

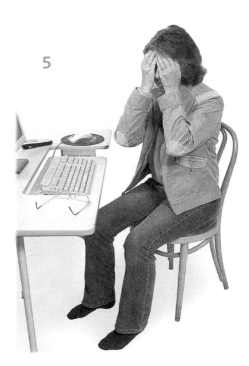

The Yoga Poses

The following are a series
of traditional yoga poses
linked together to create a
continuous flow. The first
one is very modified and
can be used by all people,
even those in a wheelchair.
The second sequence is
also modified but is more
challenging, requiring the
practitioner to be able
to stand.

Chair Sun and Moon Salutation

Step 1. Sitting tall in a chair, begin with your hands in Prayer Pose (1) over your heart. On an inhale, circle your arms out and away from your body with palms up (2), ending with your hands in Prayer Pose above your head (3). With your palms still together, exhale and lower your hands just in front of your heart (4).

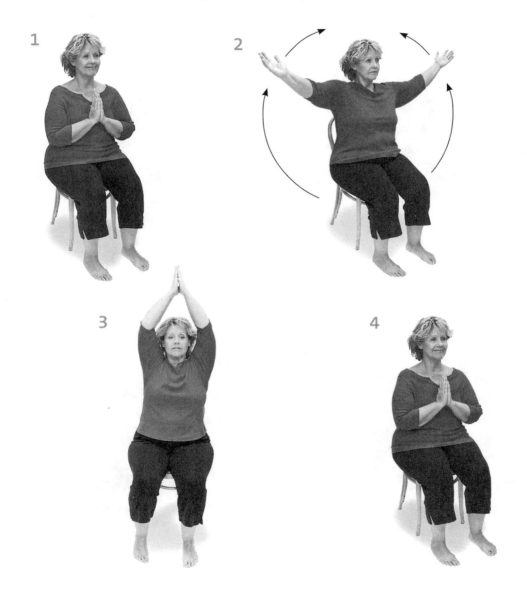

Step 2. With your palms still in Prayer Pose, inhale. On the exhale, twist your torso to the right, bringing your left elbow toward your right thigh (5). As you inhale again, return to Prayer Pose (6). On an exhale, twist your torso in the opposite direction, bringing your right elbow toward your left thigh (7). As you inhale, return to Prayer Pose (8). Exhale and release any tension.

Step 3. On your next inhale, circle your arms upward (9) until they are directly above your head to Upward Salute (10). Exhale and lower them

5

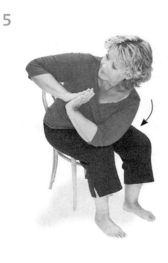

6

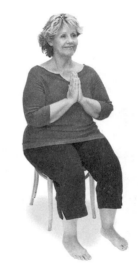

7

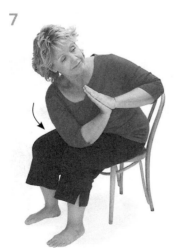

8

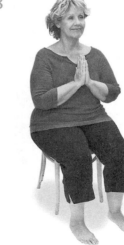

into a position just in front of you with palms facing each other and thumbs toward the sky (11). With relaxed shoulders, inhale and lift your arms to Upward Salute (12). As you exhale, bring both hands to your hips (13).

9

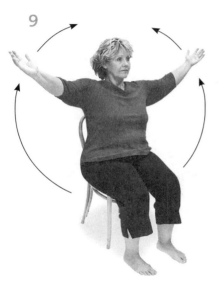

10

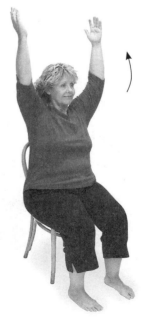

11

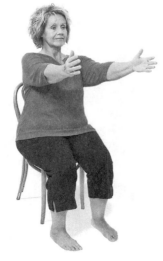

12

Step 4. On an inhale, squeeze your elbows and shoulder blades toward each other, press your chest forward, and lift your breastbone up, creating an arch in your back (14). (Imagine that you are holding a big beach ball between your elbows behind your back). On an exhale, tuck your chin toward your chest and roll your shoulders forward, rounding your back (15). Pulling the navel toward your spine will help expel old, stale air from your lungs. Inhale as you sit upright (16). Exhale and relax.

13

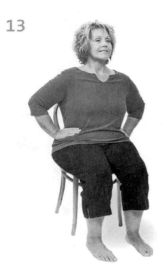

14

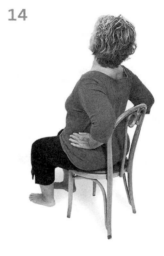

15

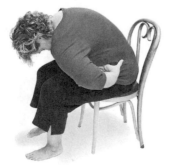

16

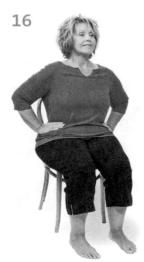

Step 5. On an inhale, circle your arms out and away from your body with palms up (17), ending with your hands in Prayer Pose above your head (18). As you exhale, lower your hands into Prayer Pose just in front of your heart (19).

Step 6. Take several breaths and, on an inhale, when you are ready, circle your arms out and away from your body with palms up (20), ending with your hands in Prayer Pose above your head (21). Keep your shoulders relaxed and away from your ears.

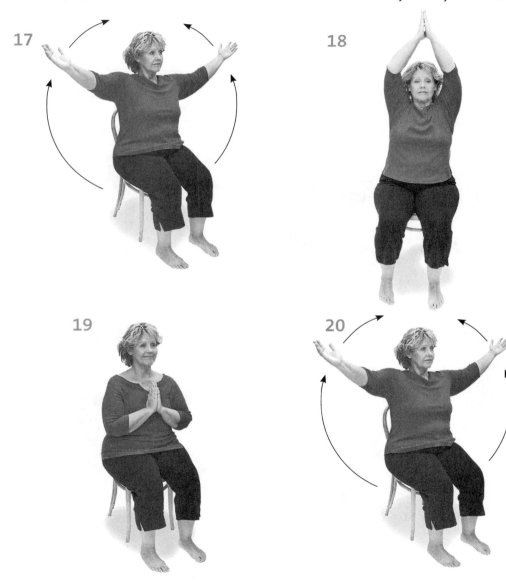

17

18

19

20

While exhaling, gently bend your upper body to the right, keeping both sitting bones and thighs firmly on the chair (22). On the inhale, return your hands to Prayer Pose above your head (23).

As you exhale, bend your upper body to the left (24). An inhale brings your body straight and your hands in Prayer Pose above your head (25). As you exhale, gently circle both outstretched arms downward around your

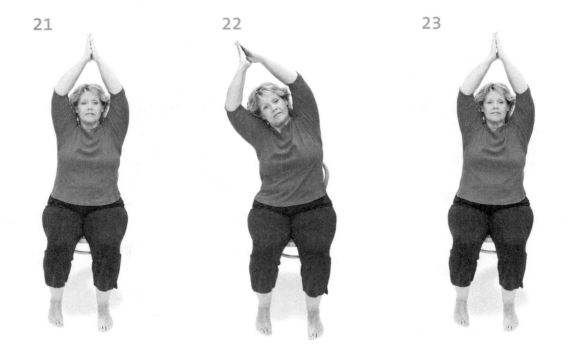

21

22

23

body, ending in Prayer Pose just in front of your heart (26).

Step 7. On an inhale, circle your arms out and away from your body with palms up (27), ending in Prayer Pose above your head. Simultaneously lift your right leg straightforward, pressing your heel away from you (28). On your exhale, return your foot to the floor while gently circling both outstretched

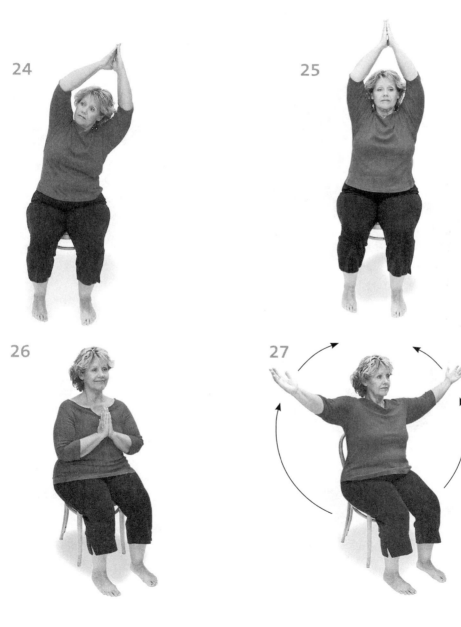

arms, ending in Prayer Pose just in front of your heart (29). Repeat this entire step lifting the left leg.

Step 8. Repeat step #7 one more time.

Step 9. Repeat step #6 again.

Step 10. On an inhale, circle your arms out and away from your body, with palms up (30), ending with your hands in Prayer Pose above your head (31). With your palms still together,

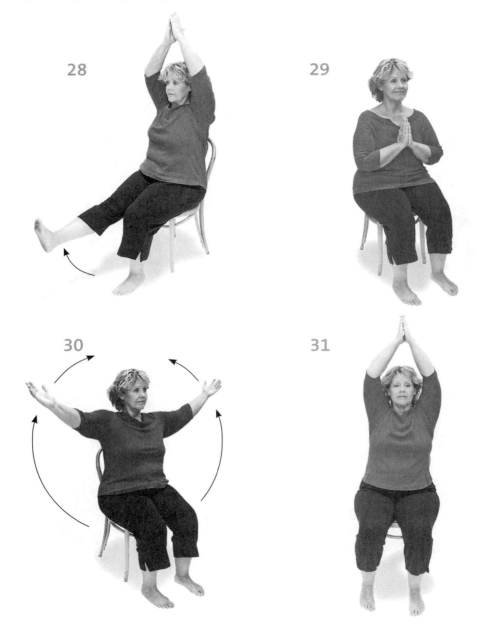

exhale and lower your hands just in front of your heart (32).

Step 11. Close your eyes, breathe normally, and listen to your heartbeat. Following several breaths, allow the backs of your hands to float to your lap (33). Take a few moments to note any sensations in your body, such as increased circulation, deeper breathing, etc. Also notice how your attitude has changed. Have you become calmer, more serene, and tranquil?

Step 12. When you are ready, slowly and gently open your eyes.

Benefits: This sequence moves your spine in six different directions. It warms up your major joints, increases your flexibility, and improves your posture while encouraging you to take fuller and deeper breaths.

Tip: The Sun and Moon sequence can even be practiced sitting in a wheelchair. It is a great activity to start your morning or to use during the day to lift your mood and boost your energy.

32

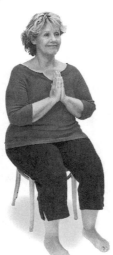

33

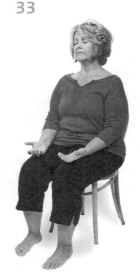

Chair-Assisted Sun Salutation

Step 1. Stand facing the chair; bring your hands to Prayer Pose just in front of your heart (1).

Step 2. Inhale and raise your arms above your head to Upward Salute (2), keeping your shoulders relaxed and away from your ears.

Step 3. On the exhale, with knees slightly bent, hinge forward at the hips (this is different from bending forward from the waist: The idea is to bend at the hips like a door hinge keeping your back flat) as far as you can comfortably go, resting your hands on the side edges of the chair seat (3).

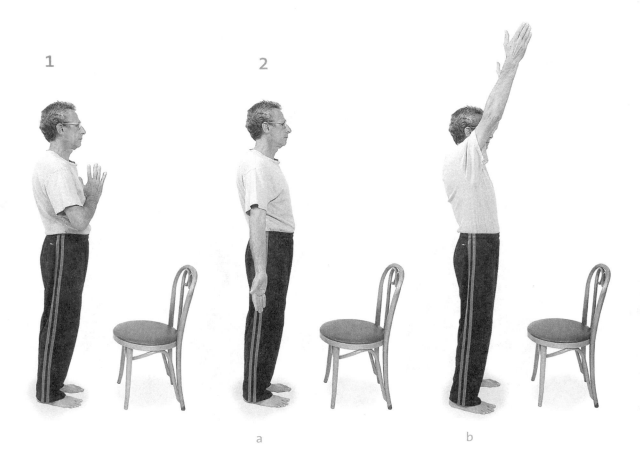

1

2

a

b

3

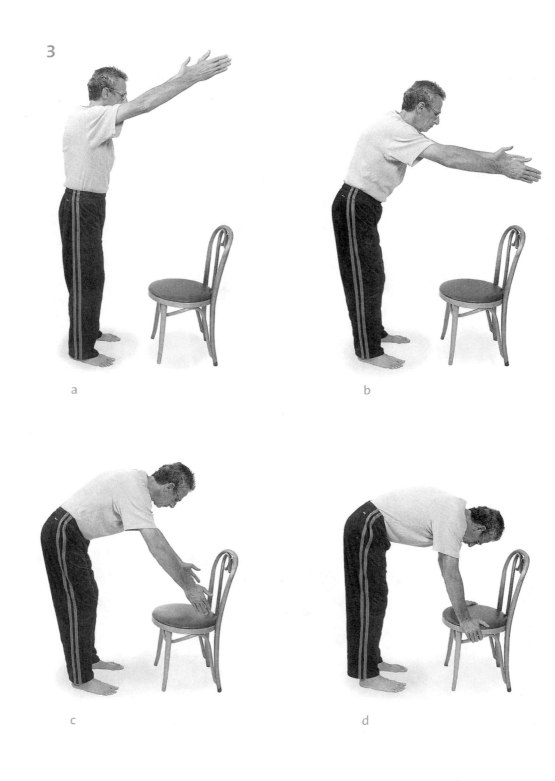

a

b

c

d

Step 4. Round your back and press the middle of your back toward the sky, tucking your chin to your chest and your tailbone toward the floor (4). You will look like a stereotypical Halloween cat. Be sure that you keep the weight of your body on your legs rather than on your hands or wrists.

Step 5. Inhale and flatten your back (5). Then exhale and step your right

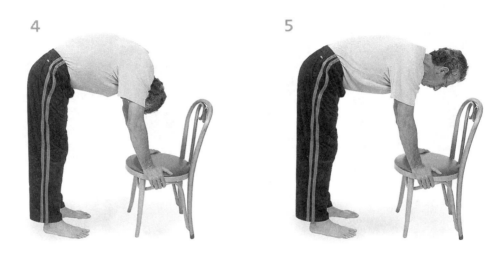

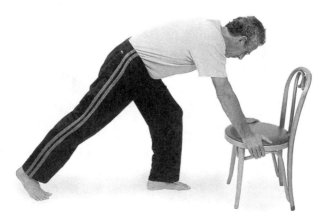

foot backward as far as you can manage while still remaining balanced (6). **Step 6.** Take another deep breath in and, on the exhale, step the left foot back to a position even with the right foot (7). Press your hips back and upward and lower your head between your arms to go into Downward-Facing Dog (8).

7

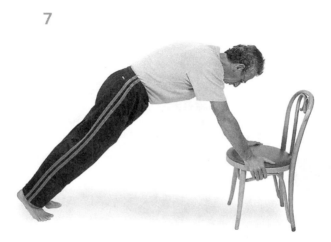

8

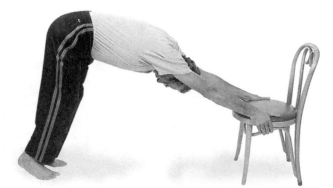

Step 7. Inhale, and move your torso forward (9), curving your hips toward the chair seat. Draw your shoulders away from your ears and invite your breastbone to move forward and upward, expanding the chest (10).

Step 8. On an exhale, press your sitting bones upward and backward toward the sky (11), lower your head between your arms and press your chest toward your thighs for Downward-Facing Dog (12).

Step 9. On an inhale, step your right foot forward into a lunge, bending the right knee so that it is directly above the ankle (13). Looking down, you should see your big toe. If not, move your knee toward your pinkie toe to prevent knee stress or injury.

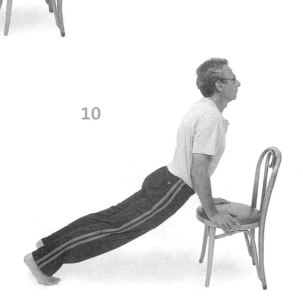

11

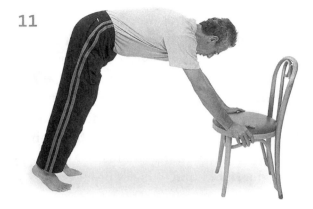

12

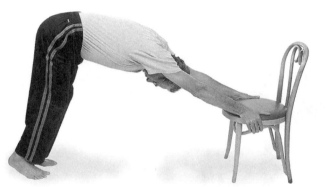

13

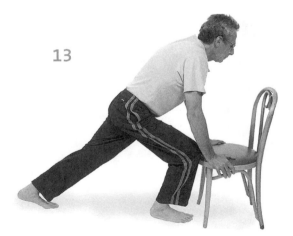

Step 10. On the next inhale, move your right hand from the edge of the chair to the top of the chair seat. Spread your fingers wide to release any pressure from your wrist. Exhale, and turn your back foot outward to forty-five degrees (14). Inhale, and lift your left arm to the sky, rotating the rib cage and chest and opening the front of your body (15).

Step 11. Slowly lower your left arm and place your hand on your left hip or your tailbone, whichever is more comfortable for you (16).

Step 12. Inhale, and raise your left arm straight upward (17) and, on the exhale, lower it and rest your hand on the side edge of the chair (18). Move your right hand to the opposite edge of the chair.

14

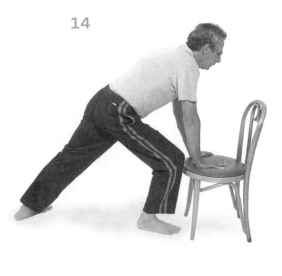

15

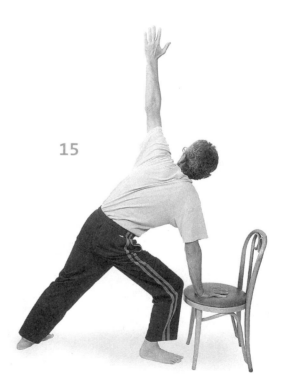

16

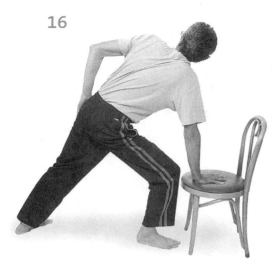

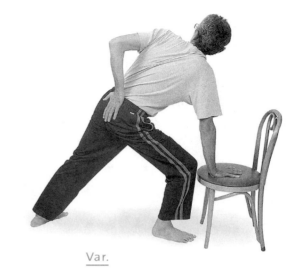

Var.

17

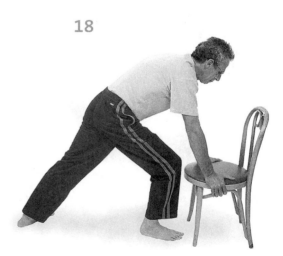

18

Step 13. Rotate your left heel so the toes are facing forward, coming back into lunge position (19).

Step 14. Take a breath in and, on the exhale, press your right foot to the floor. Step your left foot forward to meet the right, so you are in the flat back pose once again (20).

Step 15. Using the strength of your legs, press both feet to the floor. On an inhale, release the chair (21). Sweep your arms outward with palms facing

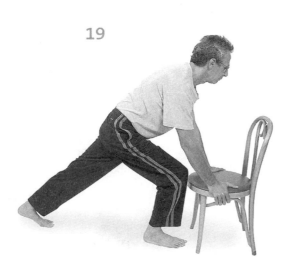

19

20

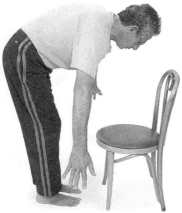

21

22

upward (22), into upward salute (23). **Step 16.** On an inhale, lift the rib cage upward and away from the hips, stretching even taller (24). On the exhale, press your hips and thighs forward, squeeze your shoulders, and create a back bend (25). Lift your breastbone upward. Looking upward is fine but do not crunch the back of your neck.

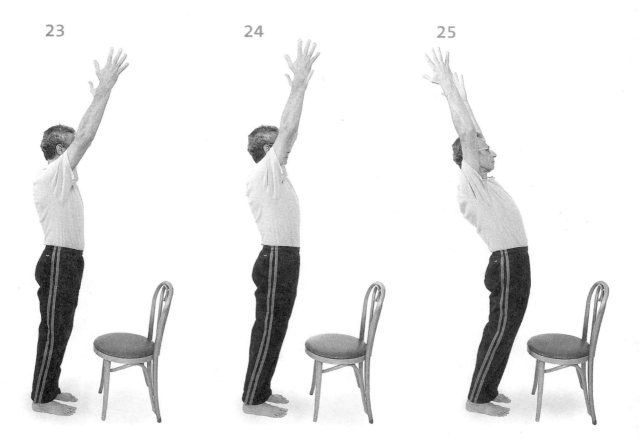

23 24 25

"I generally practice regular yoga. But while bowling recently, I twisted my back and was unable to get down onto the floor. I practiced the Chair-Assisted Sun Salutation and felt better. I was able to continue bowling and averaged 181 for the day." — Brenda

Step 17. On the next inhale, release the back bend and return to the upward salute (26).

Step 18. As you exhale, lower your hands into Prayer Pose just in front of your heart (27).

Congratulations! You have completed one half of your Sun Salutation!

Repeat the entire sequence, leading with your left foot in step #5.

Benefits: This sequence moves your spine in all directions and warms up your major joints. It will increase your flexibility and improve your posture and coordination.

Tip: Begin your day with this sequence to energize your body. Make each movement slowly, deliberately, and with awareness. Always coordinate your breath with the movement.

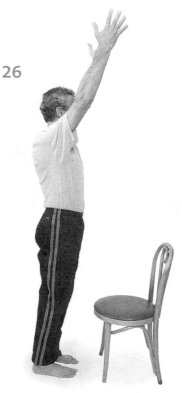

26

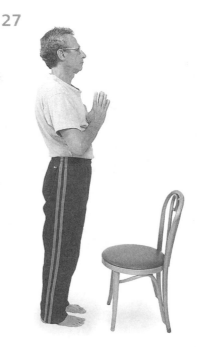

27

Shoulder-Strap Stretch

Sit tall in your chair. Hold a strap, belt, tie, or scarf with both hands at waist level in front of you. Your arms should be positioned a comfortable distance apart (1). On an inhale, raise your arms as high as you are able, keeping your fingers relaxed and your wrists and elbows straight (2). Hold the strap softly, as if it were a butterfly's wings. Although your arms are stretched,

your shoulders are relaxed. On an exhale, lower your arms to the starting point. Repeat several times, raising your arms slightly higher with each attempt. Feel the movement in your shoulder joints and visualize the joints loosening. If you are able to, bring the strap behind your head for a deeper stretch (3).

1

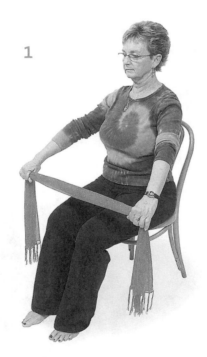

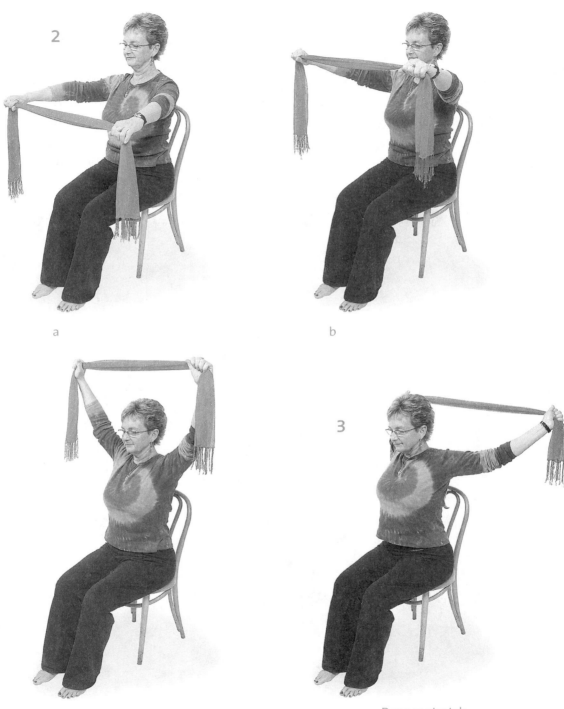

a

b

c

Deeper stretch

Benefits: This sequence stretches the arms, pectoral muscles, and torso. It allows for deeper respiration and helps prevent a hunched back.

Golfer's Tip: Warm up on the golf course! For a more relaxed swing, use one of your clubs in place of the strap to loosen your shoulders before teeing off (4).

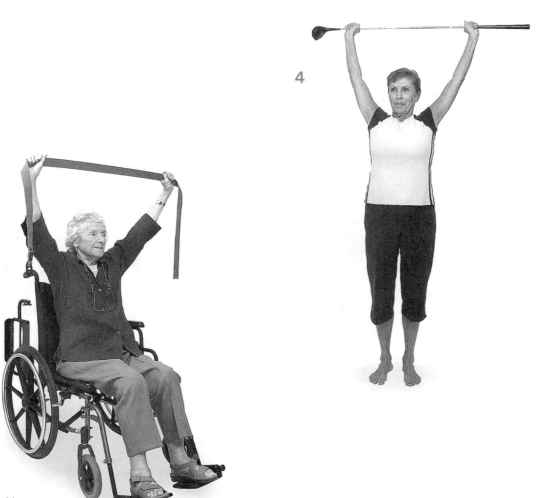

4

Var.

Shoulder Clock

Stand with your left hip 6–8 inches away from a wall. Imagine your arms are the hands of a clock. Raise your left arm to twelve o'clock (1). While breathing in and out gently, rotate your left shoulder until the palm of your hand faces the ceiling (2). On an inhale, slowly move your hand to eleven o'clock (3), then on the next inhale to ten o'clock and possibly to nine o'clock. Going any farther may hyperextend the shoulder, which is not advisable. Keep both hips straightforward. To deepen your stretch, slowly turn your toes to the right (4). After several breaths, slowly move your toes

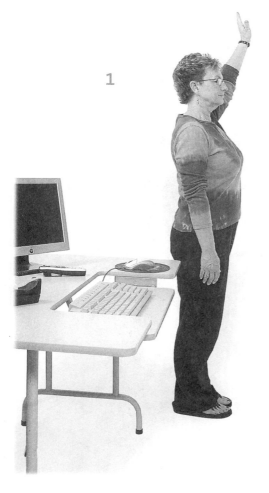

1

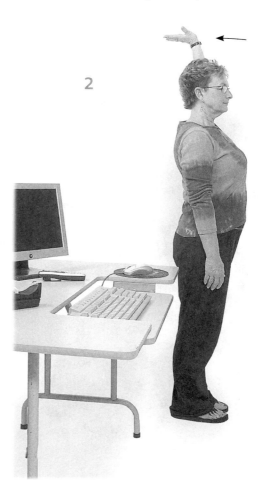

2

and your left hand back to the beginning position. Consciously allow your arm to drop forward and let it swing freely, without controlling it. Feel the difference in length between your arms and the spaciousness in the left shoulder. Turn around with your right side to the wall and repeat the sequence with your right arm and moving your hand to one, two, or possibly three o'clock.

Benefits: This pose relieves tension in the shoulders and upper back. It increases flexibility and opens the rib cage for deeper respiration.

Tip: This is a great companion to the Shoulder-Strap Stretch for relieving tension created by sitting at your desk or computer too long. Try it after any activity that causes you to hunch over, such as reading, sewing, etc.

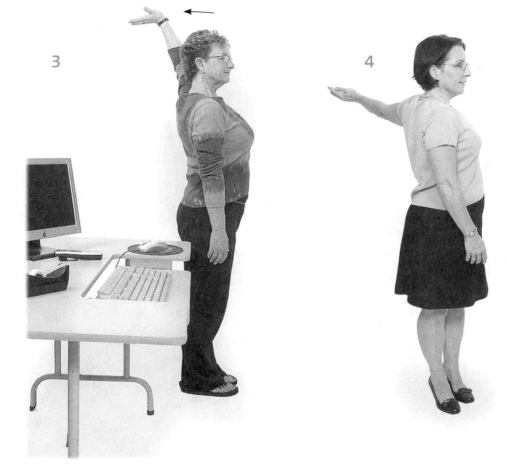

Cat/Cow Pose

Sitting tall in your chair and with your arms open, take a deep breath and press your chest forward and your shoulders backward, creating a gentle arch in your spine (1). Visualize a string at your breastbone that is pulling you gently forward and upward. Look up slightly if it is comfortable but don't crunch the back of your neck. On an exhale, tuck your chin toward your chest and roll your shoulders forward, rounding your back (2). Pulling the navel toward the spine helps expel stale air. Invite the middle of your spine to move toward the back of the chair for a deeper stretch. Keeping your chin tucked, slowly straighten your back one vertebra at a time, bringing your head up as the last movement in the exercise. Repeat several times.

Benefits: This pose incorporates two of the six movements of a healthy spine, keeping it supple and flexible. It helps open your chest and front body, promoting deeper respiration and preventing hunchback.

1

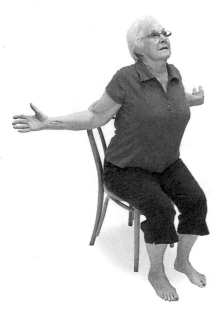

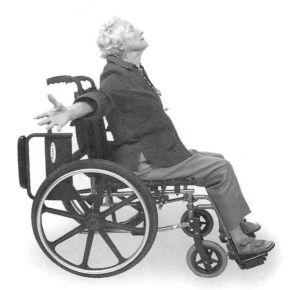

Var.

Travel and Commuting Tip: On an airplane, relieve spinal tension easily while still in your seat. Or incorporate some deep breathing into your commute as you wait for the red light to change. Holding on to the steering wheel, press your chest forward and squeeze your shoulder blades toward each other. It is guaranteed to make your ride home less stressful.

2

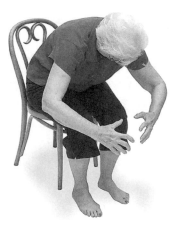

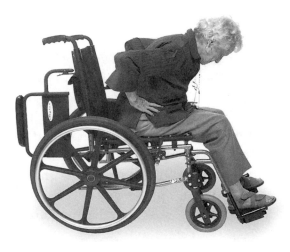

Var.

Traditional Cat/Cow Pose

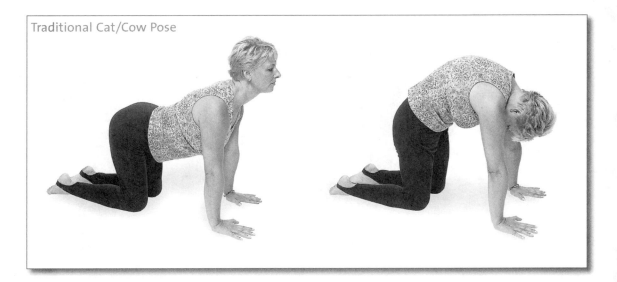

Wiggle Waggle

Place your hands firmly on a desk, kitchen counter, or other heavy piece of furniture. Bend forward at your thigh creases and walk your feet backward until your arms are straight (1). Slowly press your left hip away from your hands, simultaneously moving your right hip toward your hands by increasing the bend in your right knee (2). Keep your shoulders moving away from your ears and visualize lengthening your neck. Then press your right hip away, bend your left knee, and stretch your right side (3). Continue to breathe and repeat the movement several times. When you release the pose, slowly walk your feet forward

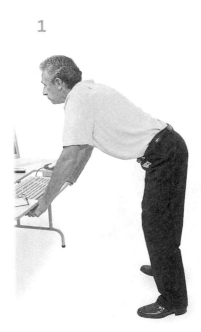

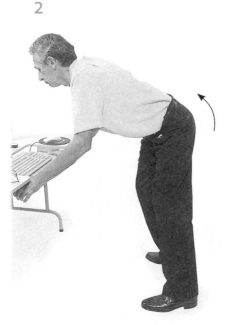

and come to a standing position with a rounded back, lifting the head up as the last movement.

Benefits: These movements release tension accumulated in your legs, hips, and torso after prolonged sitting. They stretch both sides of your body and lengthen your spine.

Tips:

- Take a break while at your desk. Several times during the day, stand up and step away from your computer. Practice the Wiggle Waggle to loosen your spine.
- If you have good balance, Wiggle Waggle can be practiced without props. Try the pose hands-free or while holding on to something with just one hand (4).

4

"I do the Wiggle Waggle while I brush my teeth in the morning. It creates a pleasant wave in my spine. It feels soooooo good after having been in bed all night." — Shirley

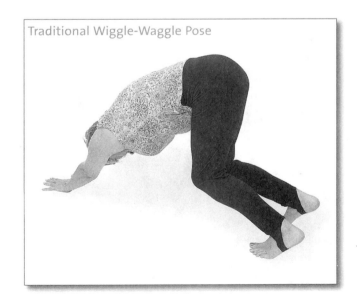

Traditional Wiggle-Waggle Pose

Child Pose/Rag Doll

Sitting tall in a chair, take a few deep breaths (1). On an exhale, tuck your chin toward your chest, press your hips backward, bend forward at the thigh creases, and hang like a rag doll with your arms dangling toward the floor (2). Allow your belly either to be sup- ported by your thighs or hang freely between your thighs. Continue to breathe. Feel the weight of your head and shoulders and let yourself relax even more deeply (3). To come up from this pose, keep your chin tucked toward your chest and roll up one

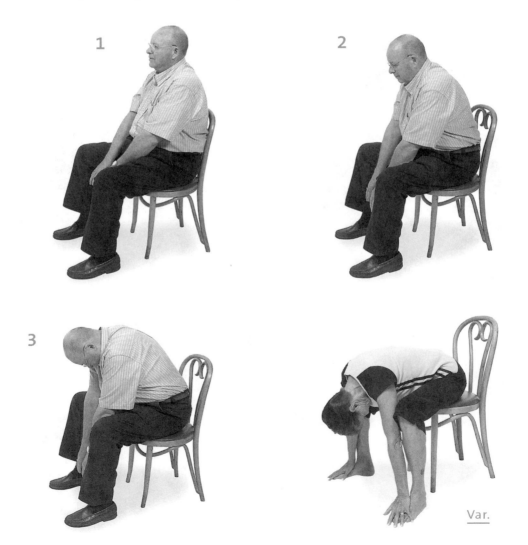

1

2

3

Var.

vertebra at a time (low back, middle back, and upper back). Finally roll your shoulders up and bring your head up last.

Benefits: Child Pose is relaxing to your nervous system and gently stretches your back muscles and your spine. It also massages your internal organs.

Tip: If you have a heart condition, place a pillow on your lap and rest your chest on it (4). Another alternative is to place a second chair in front of you (5). Stack one or more pillows on it until the height is appropriate for you. Rest your forehead on the pillows and enjoy.

4

5

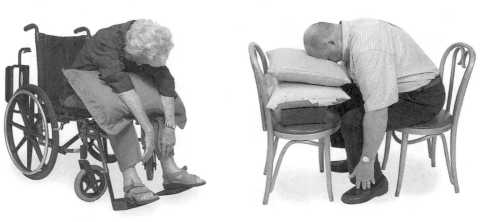

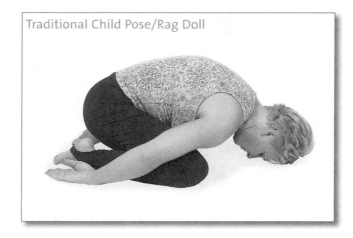

Traditional Child Pose/Rag Doll

Knee-to-Chest Pose

Sit tall in your chair. On an exhale, gently lift your left knee toward your chest, using the muscles of your leg (1). Breathe deeply. Interlace your fingers around the back of your left thigh, or just below the knee in the front of your leg. On another exhale, draw the knee even closer toward your body until you feel a pleasant stretch in your lower back (2). Your shoulders should remain relaxed and away from your ears as you continue to fill your belly with each inhale and empty your belly with

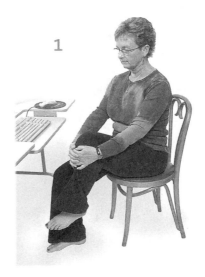

1

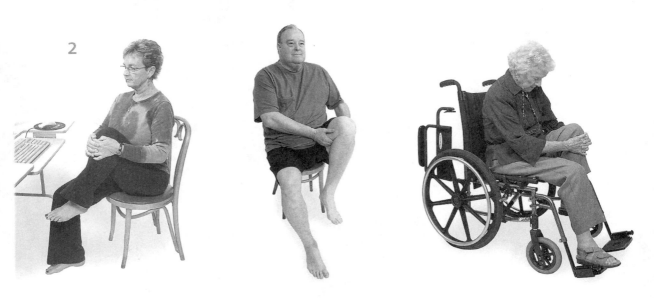

2

Var.

Var.

each exhale. Repeat several times and then switch to the right side.

Benefits: This pose will release tension in your lower back. It increases spinal flexibility and improves digestion. Yogis often refer to Knee-to-Chest as the "wind-relieving pose."

Tip: The Knee-to-Chest Pose is very easy to practice in bed (3) and is a great way to start your day. Use it often to relieve your lower back during travel. It is easily practiced even in the tight confines of an airplane seat.

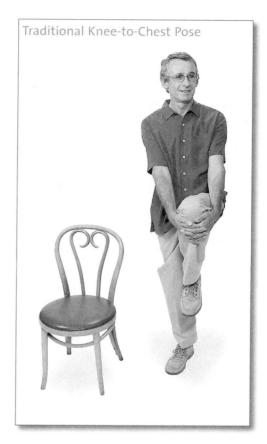

Traditional Knee-to-Chest Pose

3

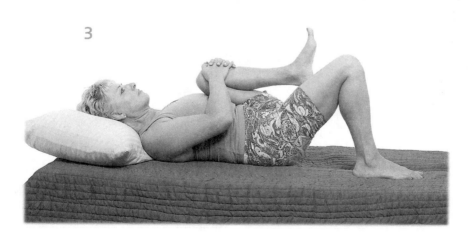

Crescent Pose

Place your right hand on the back of a chair. Stand beside the chair. On an inhale, lift the rib cage up and away from your left hip and raise your left arm to a position by your ear (1). Keep your shoulders relaxed. Press your left foot to the floor, and, on an exhale, press your left hip away from the chair, leaning your torso to the right.

Without placing any weight on the chair, create the shape of a crescent moon.

If you feel well balanced or are sitting, raise both arms into the classic Crescent Pose (2). Take several deep breaths. On an inhale, keeping the length you have created on your left side, slowly return to upright position.

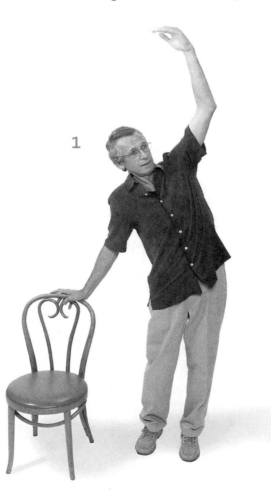

1

Walk to the opposite side of the chair and repeat the sequence to work your right side.

Benefits: This pose incorporates two of the six natural movements of a healthy spine and lengthens the spine. It stretches the side of the body and tones your arms and abdomen.

Travel Tip: When traveling or sitting for prolonged periods of time, use this stretch to relieve the scrunched-up feeling in your abdominal region.

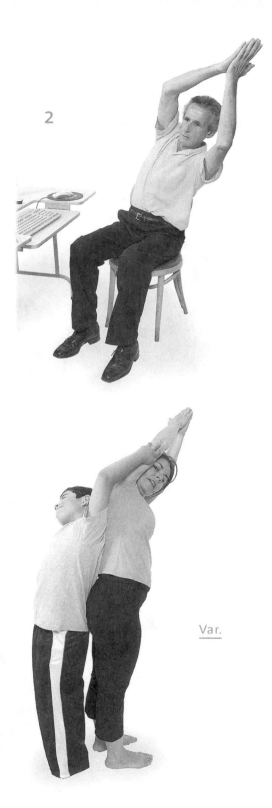

2

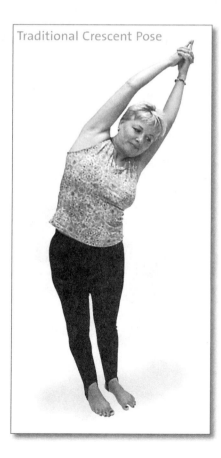

Traditional Crescent Pose

Var.

Hamstring Stretch

Stand facing the front of a chair. Place the heel of one foot on the seat of the chair with the toes of that foot pointing toward the ceiling. Plant your other foot solidly on the floor with

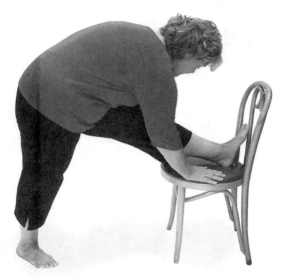

those toes pointing outward at a slight angle. With your hands resting on your thighs, lean forward, bending at the hips until you feel a pleasant stretch on the back of your elevated leg. To deepen the stretch, place the hands farther down your leg or on the seat of the chair. Take several breaths and then switch legs and repeat.

Benefits: The Hamstring Stretch increases flexibility, reduces lower back pain, and improves your posture. Cyclists and other athletes appreciate stretching the hamstrings, as this greatly reduces injuries.

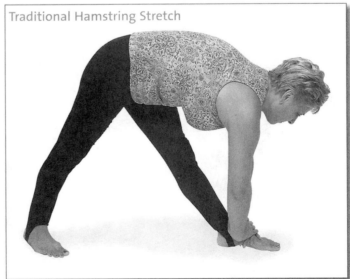

Traditional Hamstring Stretch

Tip: This stretch can be easily modified, depending on your physical needs and the environment in which you are working. You can use two chairs, a step stool, a sturdy box, or other handy items. You can also use a tie, scarf, or belt for an easier reach.

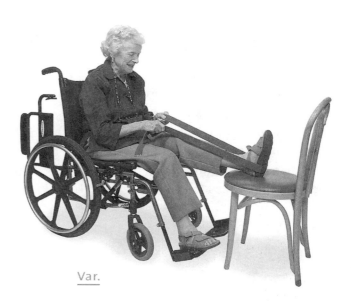

Var.

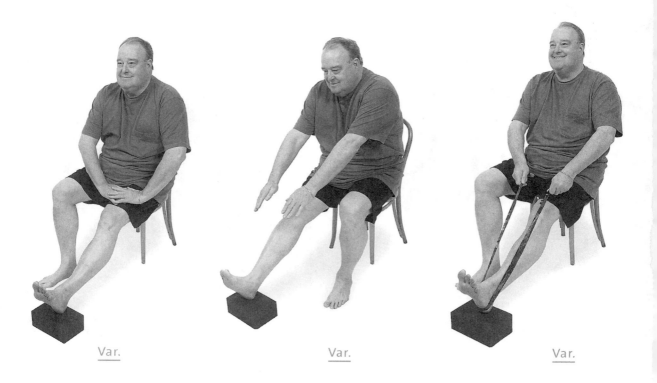

Var.

Var.

Var.

Quad Stretch/Dancer Pose

Standing next to a chair and holding on to it, bend your right knee and rest it on the seat of the chair (1). Be sure you feel balanced and are drawing the energy from the earth up through your left foot, ankle, and leg. Lean your torso forward until you feel a pleasant stretch in the quadriceps (the front of your right thigh). If this is easy for you, stand next to the chair and, while holding on to it with your right hand, bend your left knee and press it back-

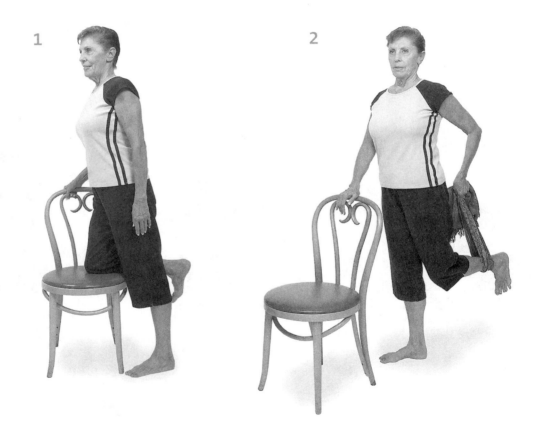

1

2

ward until you feel a similar stretch. Loop a strap, belt, or scarf around your left ankle (2). Hold on to your pant leg if you can't reach your ankle. Keep breathing and coax your knee to move farther back. If you feel well balanced, lift your left arm to a position by your ear and gently lean your torso forward (3). Hold the pose. Breathe deeply and remain focused. When you are ready, release the pose. Walk to the other side of the chair and repeat with your left knee bent.

Benefits: This pose stretches the front of your thigh and strengthens your legs, knees, ankles, and feet. It builds balance, confidence, and concentration.

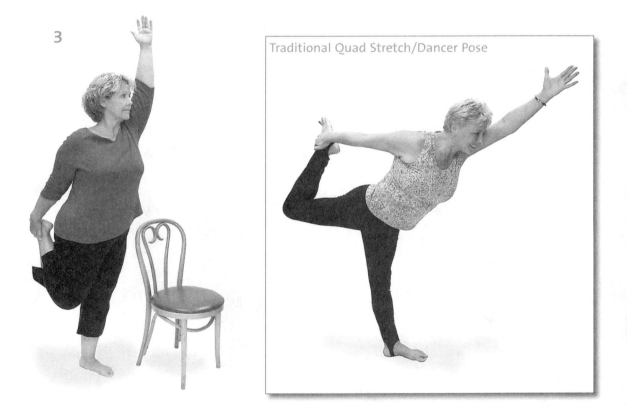

Traditional Quad Stretch/Dancer Pose

Wide-Leg Side Stretch

Sitting toward the front of your chair, open your legs as wide as possible and point your toes outward. Align your knees over your ankles to avoid knee strain. Sitting tall, hold the front edge of the chair with your left hand. On an inhale, raise your right arm toward the side of your head. On the exhale, bring your arm as close to your ear as possible. On the next inhale, lift your rib cage up and away from your hips. On the exhale, gently lean to the left. Hold the stretch for several breaths and feel the right side of your body open. If it is comfortable on your neck, look up at your hand, otherwise look down at the floor or straight ahead. If you can, roll your right shoulder toward the ceiling. When you are ready to release the pose, inhale and slowly reverse the order of the movements. Take several moments to feel the differences between the two sides and then repeat, using the opposite arm.

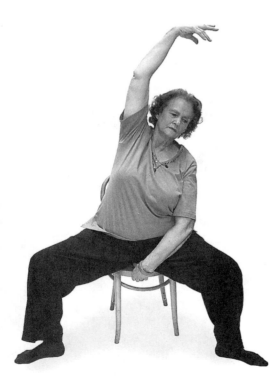

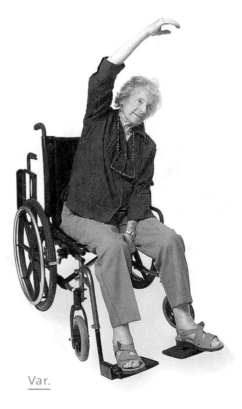

Var.

Benefits: This pose incorporates two of the six natural movements of a healthy spine into your daily routine. It stretches your thighs, opens your hips joints, and expands your rib cage.

Tip: This is a fun pose to practice with a partner. Try it seated on your bed. Your partner can help you achieve a deeper stretch, which helps reduce love handles.

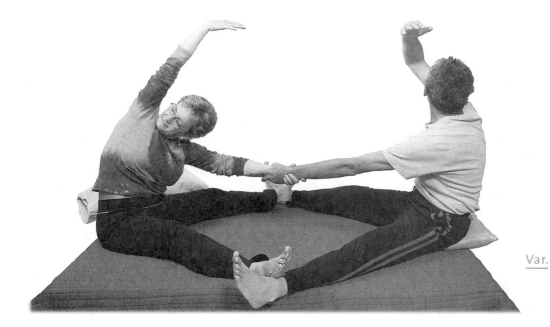

Var.

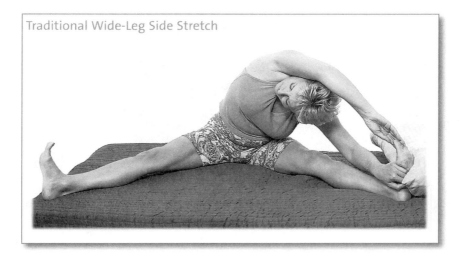

Traditional Wide-Leg Side Stretch

Downward-Facing Dog

Stand several inches in front of a chair and rest your hands on its seat. Slowly walk your feet backward and bend forward at the thigh creases. Take a deep breath and, on the exhale, bend your knees. Press your sit bones toward the wall behind you and extend your spine. Your ears should be between your arms, your chest moving toward the floor and the crown of your head facing the chair. Continue to breathe and deepen the stretch by slowly straightening your legs.

Press your sitting bones backward and upward to create an upside-down "V" shape with your body. Your shoulders are always relaxed, and your weight is supported by your legs, not the chair (1). When you are ready to come out of the pose, tuck your chin toward your chest, walk your

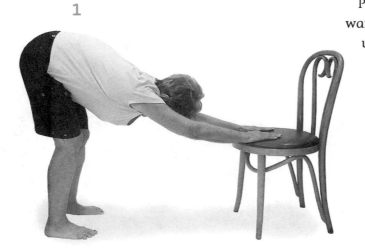

1

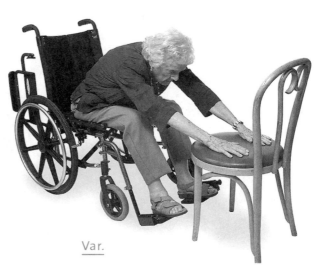

Var.

feet forward, pull your navel toward the spine and, with a rounded back, begin to stand, unrolling one vertebra at a time. If you are less flexible, begin by standing behind the chair (2); you also can use a piece of furniture or the kitchen counter.

Benefits: This pose stretches your spine and the back of your legs. It loosens your shoulders. By increasing blood flow, it helps reduce and prevent wrinkles. It aids in clearing your head, helps you focus, and quiets your mind during times of stress.

Tip: Preparing five-course meals in your kitchen can make you tired and hunched over. Rest your hands on the edge of the kitchen counter, step backward a little, and let this pose quickly rejuvenate you.

2

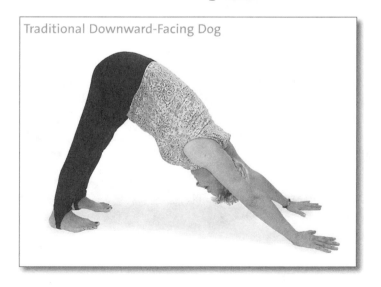

Traditional Downward-Facing Dog

Up Dog

From Downward-Facing Dog, inhale and move your torso forward, arching your back and pressing your hips and thighs toward the chair seat. Visualize a string at your breastbone that serves to gently pull it forward and upward to further open your rib cage and chest. Your shoulders should be moving toward your buttocks and away from your ears. Attempt to maintain straight legs but do not lock your knees. Take several breaths. When you are ready to release the pose, exhale and pull your navel toward your spine. Press your hips backward and lift your sitting bones up into Downward-Facing Dog. Slowly walk your feet closer to the chair and, with a rounded back, mindfully stand up.

Benefits: The Up Dog Pose tones your spine and strengthens your arms, shoulders, and wrists. It stretches your thighs and the front of your neck. It also expands your chest and stimulates your abdominal organs.

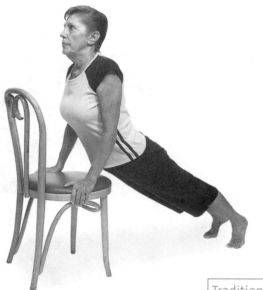

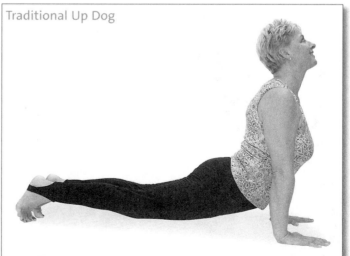

Traditional Up Dog

Archer Pose

Sit sideways with your left arm next to the back of a chair and your sitting bones toward the front of the seat. Extend your right leg as far behind you as you are able, with the sole of your foot flat on the floor and toes pointing forward and away from the chair.

Imagine you are holding a bow and arrow in front of you. On an exhale, slowly draw the bow with your right hand, swiveling your torso toward your right leg. Invite your shoulder blades to move toward your spine and allow your rib cage to expand. Hold

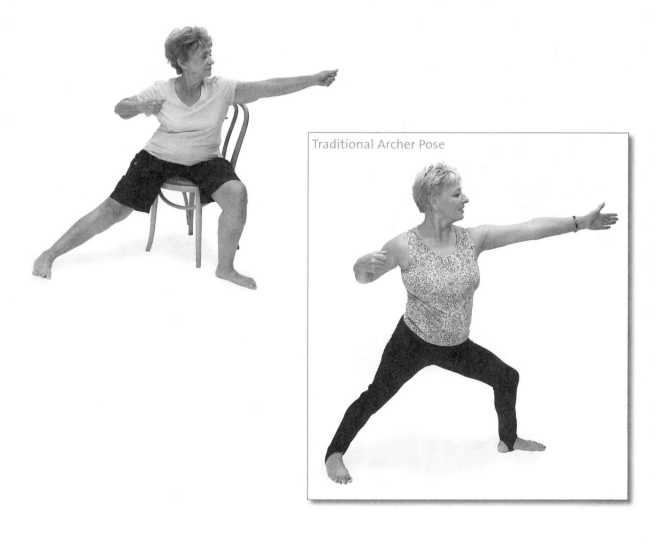

Traditional Archer Pose

the pose and breathe fully. Release and pause for a while. When you are ready, switch to the other side, extending your left leg behind you. If you have good balance, try doing the pose while standing in front of or behind the chair.

Benefits: Archer Pose helps improve balance and builds coordination and focus. It tones your arms and legs and opens your chest. It loosens your hips and shoulders.

Try this pose with a partner, friend, relative, or loved one. Stand one behind the other and simultaneously move into the pose. Partnering helps strengthen your relationship.

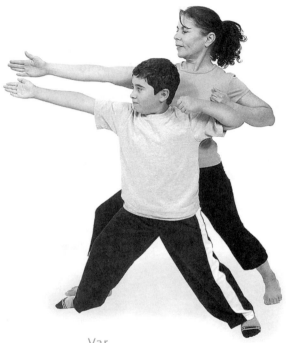

Var.

Var.

Triangle Pose

Stand next to and toward the back of the chair. Rest your right hand on the chair, with both of your feet facing forward. Rotate your right toes so they face the chair. Step your left foot sideways as far as you are able and rotate the toes toward the chair nearing forty-five degrees. Your hips will want to naturally turn toward the chair; rotate them to the left instead. On an inhale, place your left hand on your left hip. On an exhale, lean toward the chair without putting weight on it. It is fine if your right knee bends slightly. Pressing your left foot to the floor will maximize your stretch. To release the triangle, engage your leg muscles by pressing both feet to the floor, imagining you are a puppet on a string as you lift up to a full standing position. More-flexible bodies can place the hand on the seat of the chair. Stand on the opposite side of the chair and repeat the steps. This time, hold the chair with your left hand and step your right foot backward.

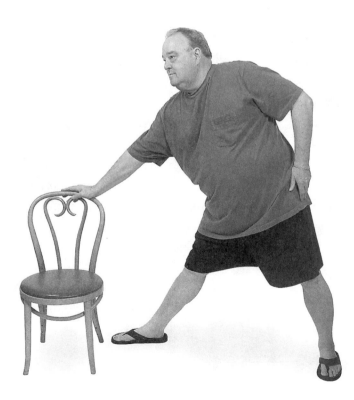

Build confidence and trust by standing in front of a partner. Simultaneously raise your left arms toward the sky as you both lean to the right, allowing your right hands to glide down your right legs and toward your ankles.

Benefits: This pose strengthens your legs and opens your side body, making space between your hips and rib cage. It moves the spine laterally and alleviates neckaches and backaches.

Tip: Before a flight or long trip, practice Triangle Pose to help alleviate sciatic nerve pain due to prolonged periods of sitting in confined spaces.

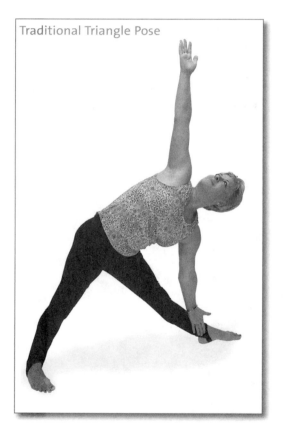

Traditional Triangle Pose

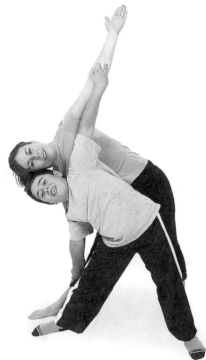

Var.

"This pose helps me a great deal during my monthly menses. Teachers have told me that because of the way I must turn my hips premenstrual symptoms are alleviated." — EP

Side-Angle Pose

Sitting forward in the chair, open your feet and legs as wide as you are able and turn both feet to the right. Slide your left foot to the side as far as is comfortable for you and swivel your hips until they both face forward. Rest your right forearm on top of your right thigh. On an inhale, lift your left arm and bring it to a position near your left ear. On the exhale, lean toward your right leg and send your breath into the left side of your body (1). If you are able, invite your raised arm to roll back slightly, which will further open your chest. If comfortable on your neck, look up toward your left hand. Take several deep, relaxing breaths and then return to the starting

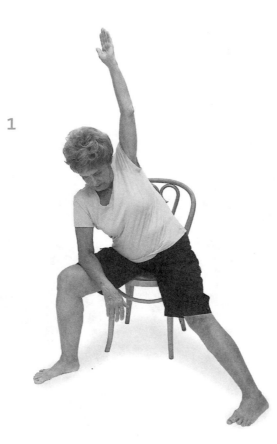

1

position. Repeat on the other side, sliding your right foot to the side and lifting your right arm.

Benefits: This pose will strengthen your legs and ankles, release tight hips, and open the chest and shoulders. It tones the arms and elongates your spine.

Tip: For a deeper stretch in the thighs, try straddling the chair backward (2). To deepen the stretch in the torso, extend the lower arm and place the hand onto the floor or onto a block next to your forward foot (3). If you are strong, try this pose standing near a chair (4).

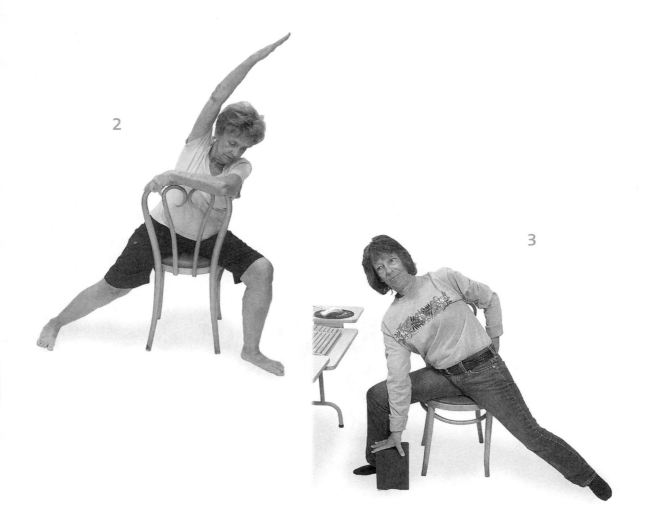

2

3

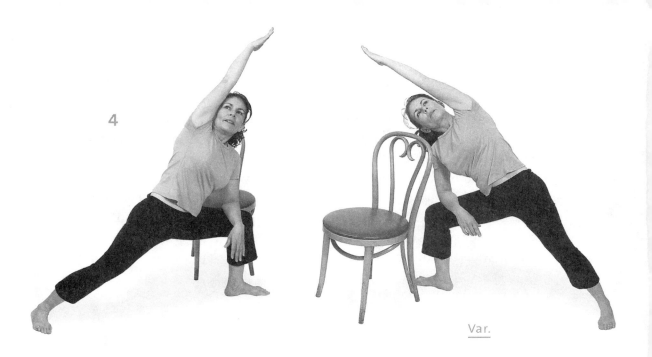

4

Var.

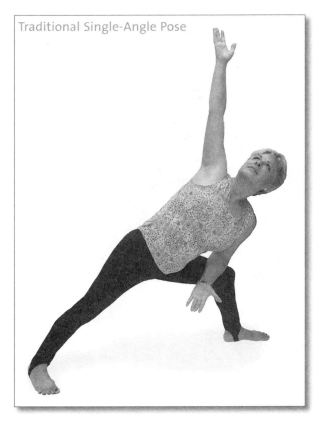

Traditional Single-Angle Pose

"The Side-Angle is one of my favorite poses. My spine feels longer, and I feel taller afterward." — Flo

Warrior I (One)

Stand behind the chair with your right hand on the backrest and your toes pointing forward. Step your left foot backward as far as you are able with your toes pointing slightly to the left. Be sure you feel balanced, and if your balance feels unstable, separate the feet a little wider. Rotate the left hip forward so that it is pointing toward the chair. Take a deep breath and, on the exhale, gently bend the right knee toward ninety degrees without allowing it to go forward of the toes. Feel your weight evenly distributed on both legs. On an inhale, raise your left arm beside your left ear (1). Keep the

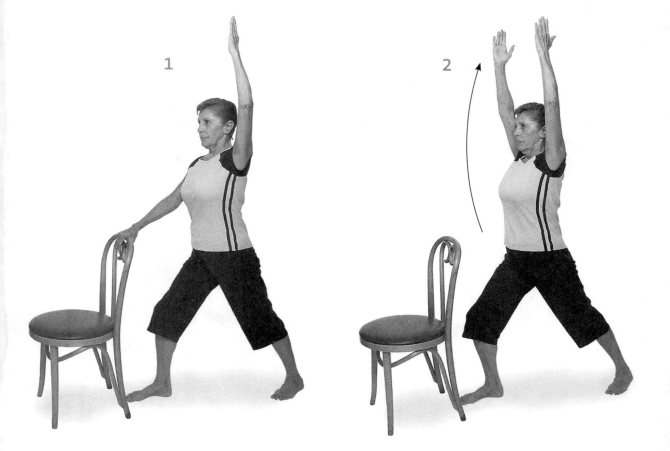

shoulders relaxed. If you are comfortable and feel well balanced, raise both arms into Upward Salute (palms apart, pictured) or Prayer Pose (palms touching) (2). After several breaths, release the hands back to the chair and, on an exhale, engage the abdominal muscles to help you step the left foot forward. Repeat on the other side, stepping the right foot backward.

Benefits: The Warrior I Pose increases flexibility in the hips, knees, and ankles. It strengthens the arms, torso, and legs and relieves shoulder and neck pain.

Office Tip: Before your important meeting or presentation, practice the three Warrior Poses to gain confidence, strength, and determination.

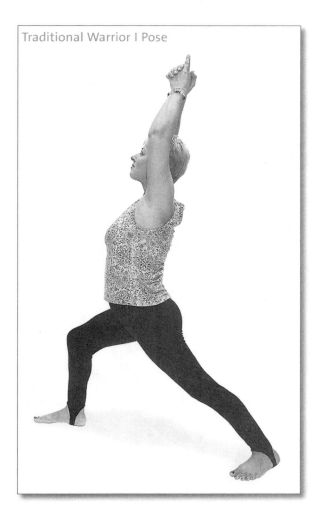

Traditional Warrior I Pose

Warrior II (Two)

Sitting forward in a chair, open your feet and legs as wide as you are able to. Turn both feet to the right. Slide your left foot to the side as far as it is comfortable and swivel your hips until they are both facing forward. Your right ankle should be directly under your knee. On an inhale, raise both of your arms to shoulder level, with your palms facing downward. Extend as if you were trying to reach both sides of the room. Keep the shoulders relaxed and softly gaze over your right middle finger (1). Hold the pose for several breaths and release it when you are ready. Sit quietly. In your mind, observe the space you have created through your chest and rib cage. Feel the openness of your hips and thighs. Repeat this pose on the other side, with the left foot and leg forward. The well-balanced person may want to try standing behind the chair (2).

If this is easy for you, try the pose hands-free by standing behind a chair, knowing the chair is available if you need it to help maintain your balance (3).

Benefits: The Warrior II Pose increases flexibility in your hips and lower joints. It strengthens your ankles, legs, and thighs, works your shoulders, and energizes your arms.

Tip: When you need help getting through the day, practice the Warrior II Pose and affirm positive thoughts, such as: "I am peaceful," "I am strong," etc....

Traditional Warrior II Pose

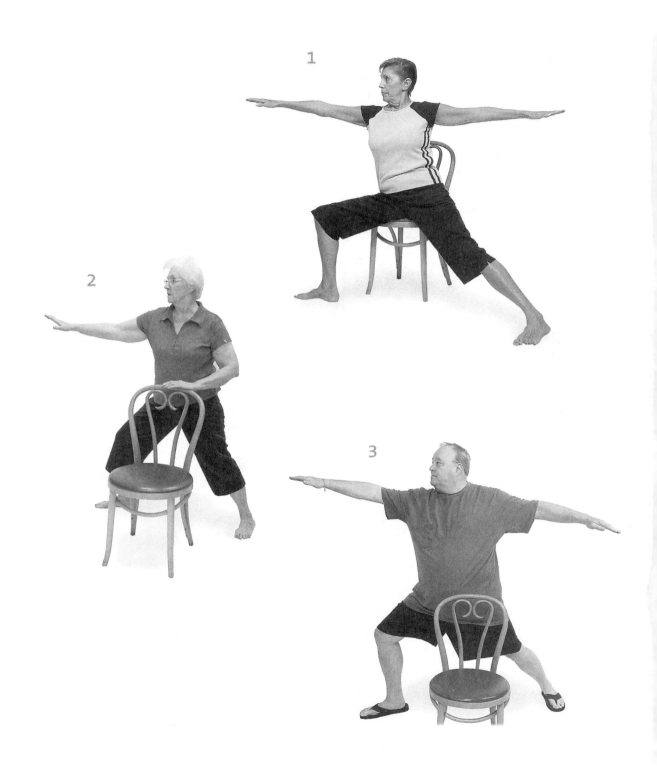

1

2

3

Warrior III (Three)

Stand behind the chair and place your right hand on the back of the chair. Step the left foot backward with the toes pointing slightly forward and outward. Pressing your right foot to the floor, slowly lift your left leg, extending it backward and upward as high as you are comfortable. This action will enable your torso to move forward and your body will form a "T." Keep the standing leg as straight as possible without locking your knee (1). Extending your left arm near your left ear will help to lengthen your spine (2). Take as many breaths as you like and when you are ready, slowly lower your arm to your side. Then gently lower your left foot to the floor. On the exhale, press the right foot to the floor. Pull your navel toward your spine and step your left foot forward to meet the right.

Repeat on the other side, stepping backward with the right foot.

This pose can also be adapted to do at work using the support of a table (3).

Benefits: The Warrior III Pose strengthens your legs and helps them become shapelier. It may relieve calf muscle cramps, tone the abdominals, and promote balance and concentration.

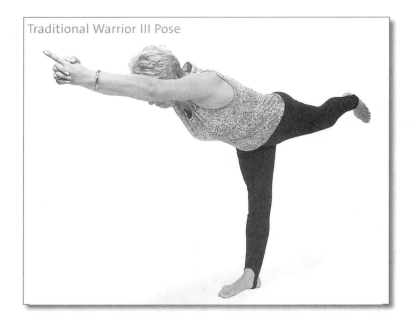

Traditional Warrior III Pose

Tree Pose

Stand tall next to a chair, holding the back-rest if needed. Ground your feet and draw the energy up from the earth. When you are ready, bring your right foot to your left ankle. You may keep your toes on the floor or you can raise them slightly. If this is too simple, raise your foot to just below or above your knee. More flexible and well-balanced practitioners may bring their foot upward to their inner thigh. As long as you feel balanced, you can let go of the chair and bring your hands into Prayer Pose just in front of your heart or above your head. Modify this by bringing just one arm upward while you hold the chair with your other hand. Invite your tailbone to move gently toward the earth and the crown of your head toward the heavens. Keep your shoulders relaxed and your chest open. Invite

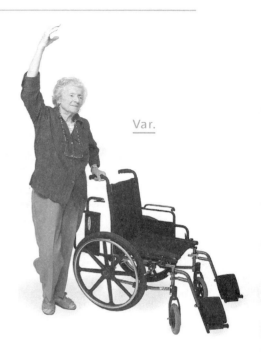

Var.

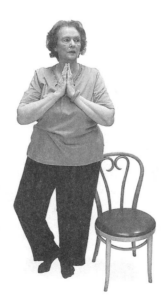

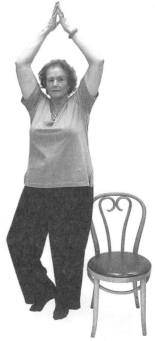

your breastbone to lift slightly. Take several breaths as you imagine the roots of your feet growing deeper into the earth. Hold this position for a few seconds. Eventually, aim toward holding the pose for one minute. Walk to the other side of the chair and repeat, with your left foot on the floor and the right foot touching the left ankle.

Benefits: Studies have shown that standing on one leg several minutes per day helps build bones and prevents osteoporosis. Tree Pose helps your balance, encourages concentration, and strengthens your legs, ankles, and feet.

Golfer's Tip: Next time you are on the golf course waiting your turn, strike a Tree Pose, using your golf club as a prop.

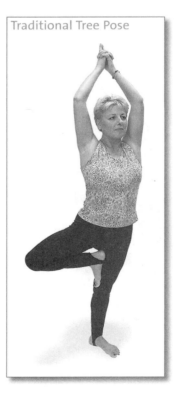

Var.

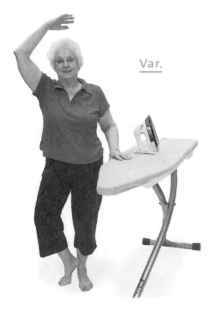

Var.

"Practicing Tree Pose improved my balance so much that I can now stand on one foot without having to hold on to something—a feat I could not achieve earlier, due to peripheral neuropathy." — Neil

Traditional Tree Pose

Chair Pose

Stand in front of a chair as if you were ready to sit in it. Let your feet be hip-width apart, your arms straight-forward, and your palms facing each other. Bend your knees just a little as if you were about to be seated. Then with each small breath, bend your knees a little deeper in small increments. Eventually, the backs of your thighs will touch the front of the chair (1). Finally, gently lower yourself onto the chair. Visualize yourself about to sit on an egg that you don't want to break. Rest. To stand, first engage your leg and thigh muscles by pressing both feet to the floor. Take a deep breath. Pull your

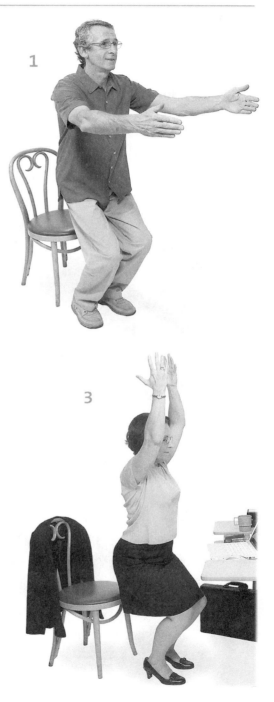

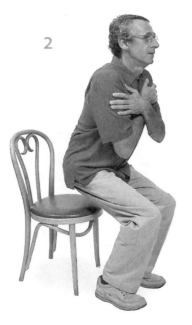

navel toward the spine to protect your lower back and begin to slowly stand up. Your legs and abdominal muscles should be doing the work rather than your back. To challenge yourself, try the pose with your arms crossed over your chest (2) or above your head (3).

Benefits: Chair Pose strengthens your feet, ankles, calves, thighs, and gluteal muscles.

Tip: Practice this pose daily, and you will soon find you can get up from the sofa and the toilet with greater ease. This is also a fun pose to practice with a partner (4). You can use each other as leverage to slightly intensify the exercise.

4

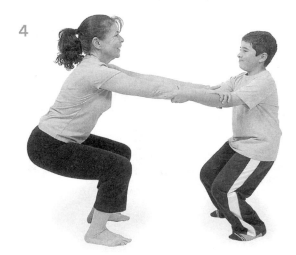

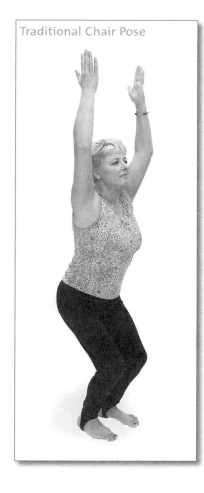

Traditional Chair Pose

"Before I started chair yoga, I had a difficult time getting out of a booth at a restaurant. I was embarrassed, so I would request to be seated at a table instead. I don't have to do that anymore because my legs have become much stronger and my back does not hurt." — Alyce

On-the-Bed Twist

Lying comfortably on your bed, exhale and bring your left knee toward your chest. Take several deep breaths, filling your lungs to their capacity, and then exhale fully, releasing all stale air. When you are ready, slowly move the bent knee across your body, keeping both shoulders firmly positioned on the bed. Continue to breathe and feel the spiral created in your spine. To deepen the twist, gently coax your knee closer to the bed by placing your hand on your thigh. Experiment by moving your knee closer or farther away from your torso to feel the spiral traveling higher or lower on the spine.

If your neck allows it, turn your head in the opposite direction. Hold the pose as long as it feels comfortable and then slowly release it. When you are ready, repeat the pose, using your right knee.

Benefits: Twists aid in digestion and elimination; they also remove toxins and help release back tension. They squeeze and soak the spine, bringing fresh, clean energy to stagnant areas.

Tip: Twists are about letting go of physical and emotional tension. When you are feeling anxious, close your eyes, twist, let go, and simply breathe. This is a fun pose to try with a partner.

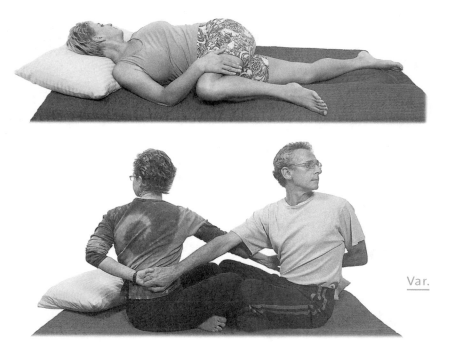

Var.

Seated Twist

Sitting tall in your chair, take a deep breath and lengthen your spine. On the exhale, gently twist your torso to the right, beginning with your lower back, then your middle, and then your upper back. Finally turn and look over your right shoulder. Never force the twist. If you wish for a deeper twist, place your hand or arm on the back of the chair for additional leverage (1). Take several deep, cleansing breaths. When you feel ready to release, exhale and slowly unwind the twist, bringing your head forward first, then your

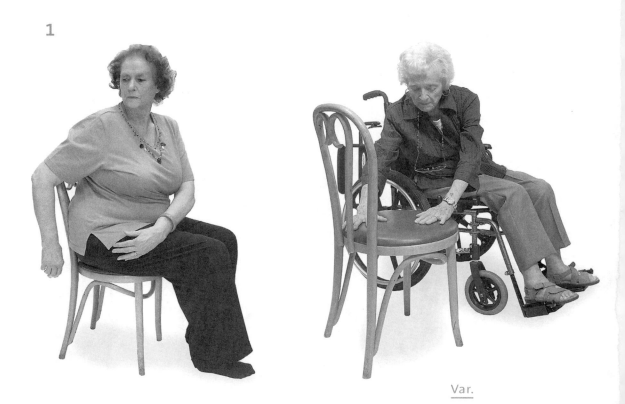

1

Var.

upper back, then your middle back, and lastly your lower back. If you are more flexible, you may wish to lower your left hand toward the floor on the outside of your right leg and raise your right arm to the ceiling (2). A fun option is to straddle the chair backward. Place your left hand on the backrest and your right hand on the seat behind you (3). Use leverage to deepen the spiral.

Benefits: Twists keep your spine flexible. They massage your internal organs and aid the body in detoxifying. Twists also help elimination.

Travel Tip: On an airplane, hold the armrest as you slowly twist—first to one side and then the other—to aid digestion and relieve travel anxiety. This pose is fun to practice with a partner in chairs or on the bed.

2

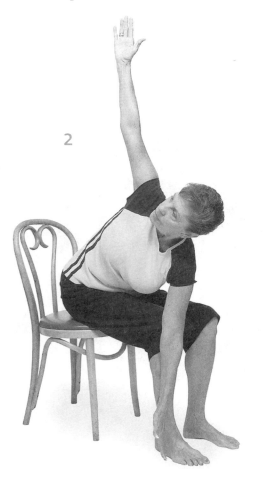

3

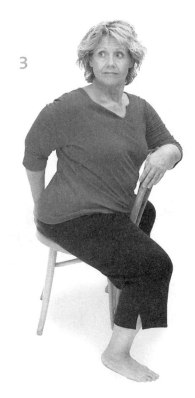

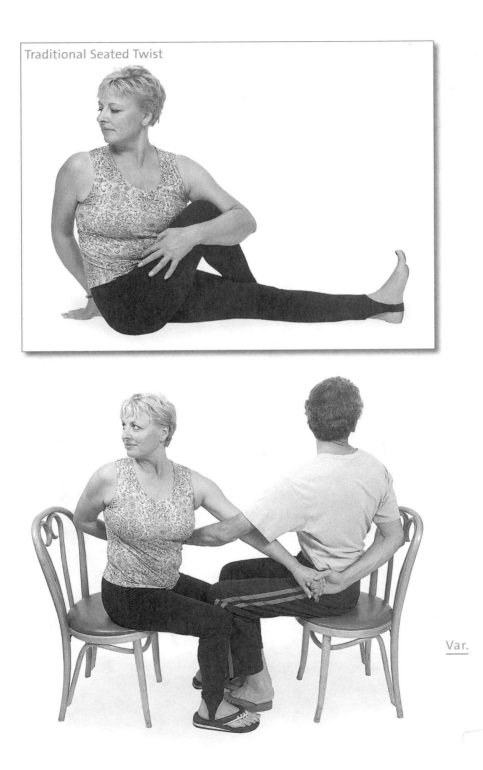

Traditional Seated Twist

Var.

Standing Twist

Stand with your right side next to a wall with a stool in front of you (1). Step your right foot onto the stool (2). Be sure you feel balanced. If you are not, make any necessary changes to the placement of your left foot until you are steady. On an inhale, lengthen your spine and tuck your tailbone slightly toward the floor. Place your hands on the wall and gently begin to move first your navel, then the rib cage, then the chest, and finally your shoulders toward the right. Simultaneously, move both hands along the wall and to the right (3). To deepen the spiral of your spine, press your hands

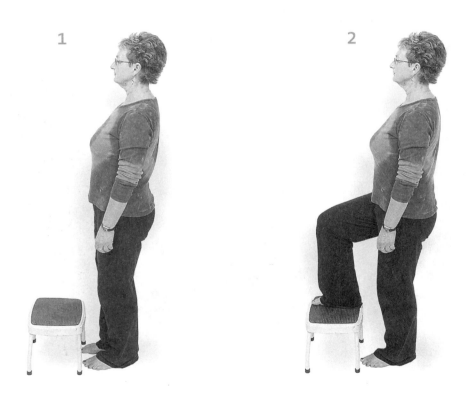

1

2

to the wall, using slightly more pressure. Stay in the pose as long as you feel comfortable and then release it by tracing the steps backward. Take a few deep, cleansing breaths before you walk to the other side of the stool and place your left foot onto it. Then repeat the same steps on the opposite side, walking your hands toward the left.

Benefits: Twists bring fresh, clean energy to your spine and aid in detoxification of your internal organs.

Office Tip: Prolonged sitting at your desk is hard on your spine. Take a break every couple of hours. You can use a chair to step on, as long as it does not have wheels or rollers on it.

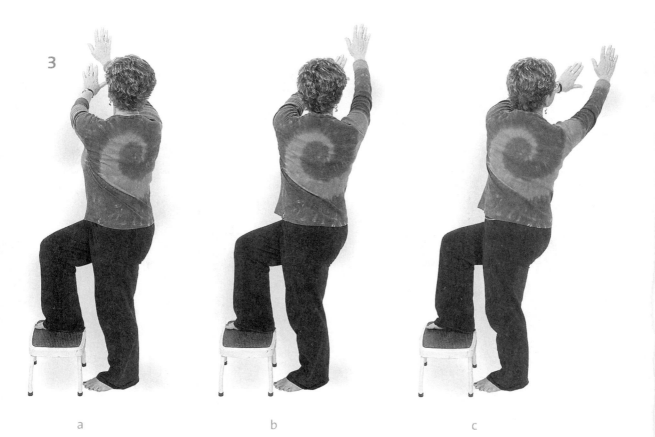

3

a   b   c

Golfer's Tip: Warm up your swing on the golf course. Stand erect holding your golf club and initiate the twist at your lower back. Visualize your spine as a spiral staircase as you twist further up the body.

For partners: Stand facing your partner. Wrap your left arm around your back, and with your left hand, hold your partner's right hand. Your partner does the same. Each partner then twists to the left, which makes them face in opposite directions. They then switch arms and repeat the twist to the right.

Var.

Var.

Sciatic Stretch Sequence

On a bed, while lying comfortably on your back (1), place a strap (towel, scarf, or belt) around the heel of your right foot (2). Gently holding the strap with both hands, lift and straighten your leg toward the ceiling (3). Press the heel away from you until you feel a pleasant stretch in the back of your leg. Holding the strap with your right hand, lower the leg as far to the right

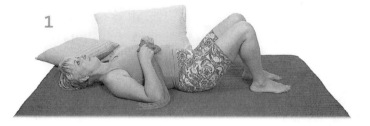

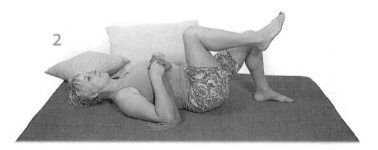

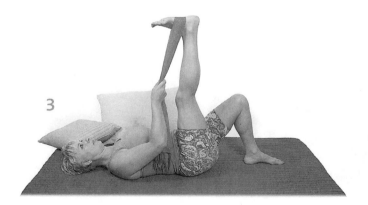

as is comfortable for you, keeping both shoulders and your left hip on the bed (4). On an exhale, slowly raise your leg back toward the ceiling again (5). Hold the strap with your left hand and lower your leg across your body to the left as far as you are able (6). Both shoulders should remain firmly on the bed, however, this time the right hip will rise off the bed. You will feel the stretch where you need it the most—possibly in the buttocks, hips and/or lower back. On an exhale, again slowly raise your leg toward the ceiling (7). Bend your knee, release the strap, and hug your thigh to your chest. Continue breathing. Slowly straighten your leg and let it rest on the bed. Notice the difference between the two sides of your body. Repeat the same sequence using your left leg.

4

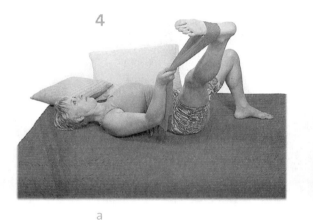

a

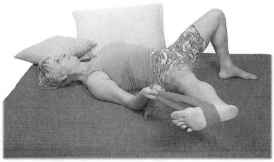

b

5

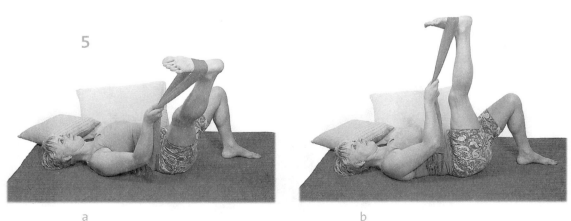

a

b

Benefits: This sequence stretches your legs, opens your hips, and releases tension in the lower back. It also relieves the sciatic nerve.

Travel Tip: When going on a trip that requires being seated for long periods of time, use this sequence before and after travel to help prevent sciatic pain.

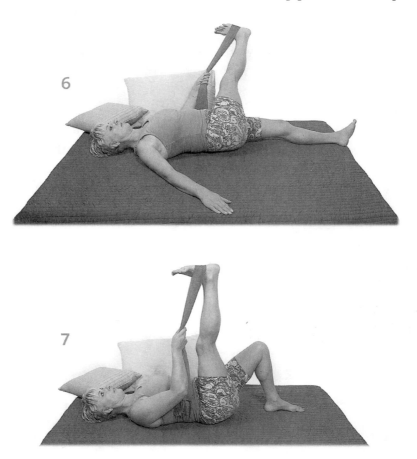

"Learning the Sciatic Stretch has relieved much of the pressure on that nerve and has helped ease the pain and numbness in my legs. I do not take pain medicine, and I am able to get around and do things that I could not have done a few years ago." — Rosemary

Cobbler Pose

Sitting tall in one chair, rest both your feet and lower legs on the seat of another chair. Slowly bring the soles of your feet together at arm's length, letting your knees bend outward like butterfly wings (1). Without strain, invite your knees to open more fully toward the floor. Take a few breaths and, on an inhale, lengthen your spine. On an exhale, press your hips and thigh creases backward and, with a straight spine, bend forward, allow-ing your chest to move toward your feet (2). Continue to breathe. Each inhale gives you an opportunity to further lengthen your spine. Each exhale allows you to deepen the pose by moving deeper into your stretch. Release the pose by rounding your back and rolling up one vertebra at a time. Then, using your palms, gently help both of your knees up and slowly rest one foot at a time on the floor.

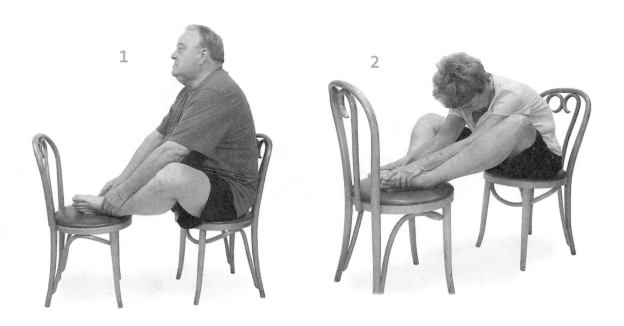

Benefits: This pose opens your hips and thighs. It stretches your back and strengthens your legs and ankles. It also massages your internal organs.

Tip: The less-flexible body can try this pose on the bed or chair using one leg at a time (3). Also try wrapping a strap, belt, or scarf around your feet (4).

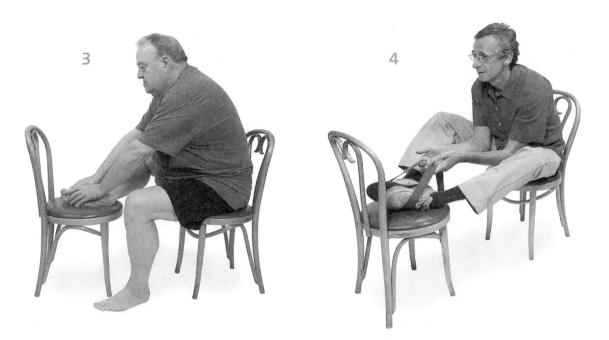

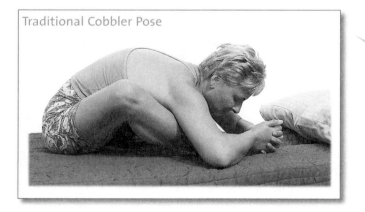

Traditional Cobbler Pose

"This pose has helped lessen the pain in my hips, and I can much more easily bend over to pick up things from the floor." — Neil

Rock the Baby, or Cradle Pose

Sitting tall in your chair, lift your right knee, clasp your hands around your shin, and hug your leg to your chest. Hold for several breaths. On an exhale, release your left hand and place it under your right ankle. Lift your foot above and across your left thigh and raise it up as high as you are able while cradling your right knee in your right hand. Gently rock your hips side-to-side as if you were rocking a baby.

For a deeper stretch or for those who are more flexible, cradle the foot in the crook of left elbow and the knee in the crook of the right. Keep your

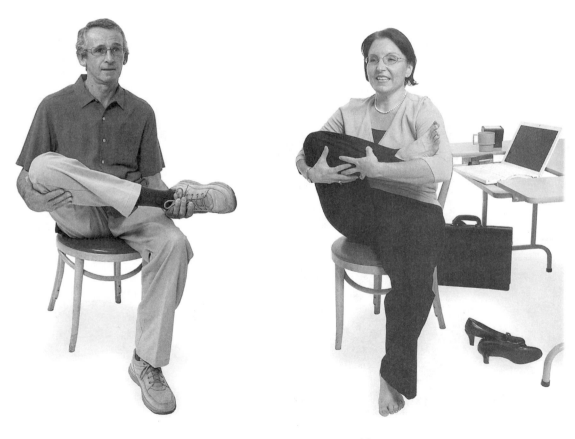

Var.

spine straight and breathe deeply into the stretch. Once you release the pose, take a moment or two to notice the differences between the side you have stretched and the side you have not yet stretched.

Repeat with other leg.

Benefits: This pose gently opens and releases tight hips. It massages the lymph nodes and stretches your legs and ankles. It also is effective for stretching the sciatic nerve.

Office Tip: Practice this pose to relieve tension in the hips and lower back when you have been sitting at your desk for a long period of time.

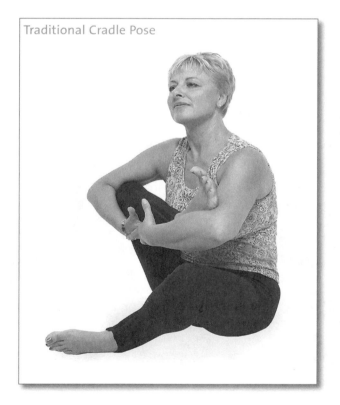

Traditional Cradle Pose

Seated Pigeon Pose

Sitting forward on a chair, rest your right ankle over your left thigh (1). Flex your right foot and spread your toes. Interlace your fingers behind your left thigh, engage your abdominal muscles, and gently lift your left leg toward you (2). As your left knee moves toward your torso, using your right elbow, coax your right knee toward the floor. Experience the opening in your right thigh and hip crease.

If you are unable to lift your left leg, simply keep your foot on the floor and only coax the right knee toward the floor (3).

For a deeper outer hip stretch, lean forward at the thigh creases. Press your torso toward your thighs (4).

Add a twist to release the spine. Place your right hand on your right ankle or foot. Hold the chair seat with your left hand and twist your torso to

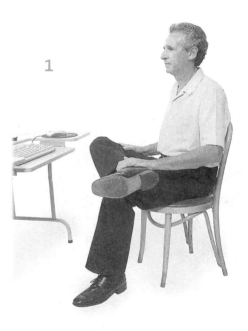

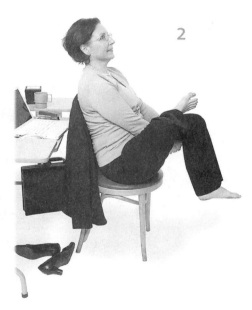

the left (5). Deepen the intensity of the twist by holding the chair back instead of the seat. Repeat the same with the other side.

Benefits: This pose opens your hips and keeps your knees and ankles flexible. When you lean forward, the spine is elongated, and the outer hips receive a deeper stretch. When you incorporate a twist, you are also squeezing your internal organs to aid digestion.

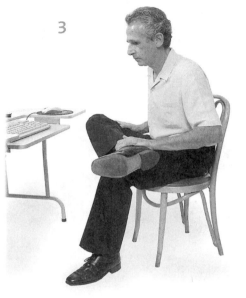

3

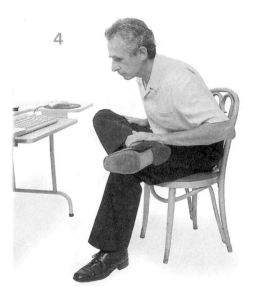

4

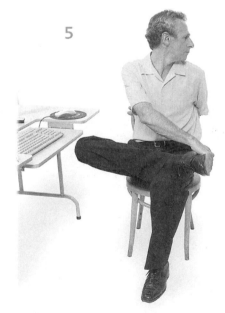

5

Travel Tip: Stretching the calves and hips helps your blood circulation to avoid deep vein thrombosis (DVT) on long flights or automobile trips. Practice the first part of this pose on the bed as soon as you arrive at your destination.

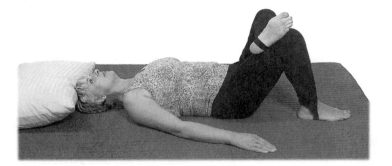

Var.

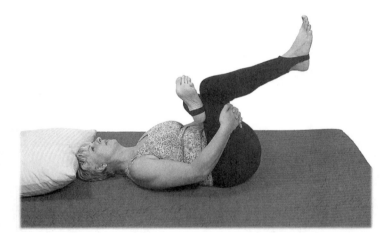

Var.

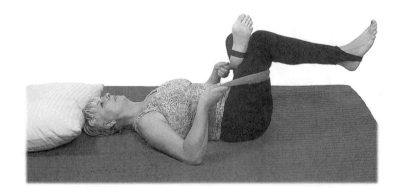

Var.

Pigeon Pose

Facing a chair, place the side of your right calf on the seat. Attempt to create as close to a ninety-degree angle as possible by placing the foot as close to the back of the chair as you are able. (The ideal ninety-degree angle will help prevent injury to the knee joint.) While holding on to the back of the chair, extend your left leg as far behind you as possible, keeping the toes or ball of the foot on the floor (1). Try lowering your hips toward the seat of the chair. If you are more flexible and feeling balanced, release the hands from the chair, press the chest forward, stretch your arms behind you, and lean into a comfortable back bend (2). Take a few breaths and, when you are ready, mindfully reverse the process. Hold on to the

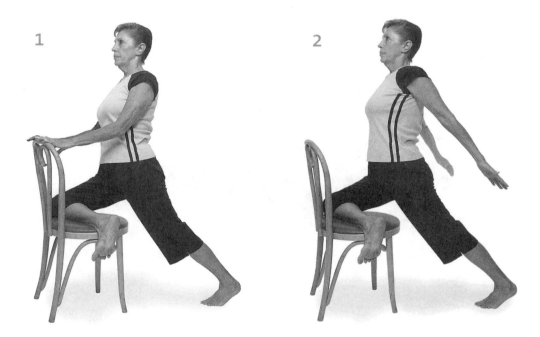

chair, release the right leg, and slowly stand up. Feel the openness of your hips and then switch to the left side.

Benefits: This pose opens your hips and stretches your groin muscles. It keeps the knees and ankles flexible. It tones your legs and increases lower-body vitality.

Tip: The Pigeon Pose is an excellent exercise for opening the hips further following the Cradle Pose (see page 106).

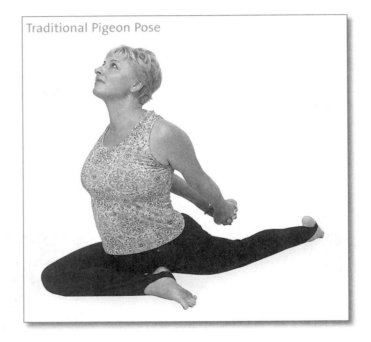
Traditional Pigeon Pose

Lumberjack Pose

With a straight back and your feet as far apart as you can, sit forward in your chair. Clasp your hands above your head, with your arms next to your ears, and take several deep breaths. Energetically breathe out through your mouth, fold forward, and allow your arms to swing as if you were to chop wood with an ax. Let your arms swing at will; try not to control them. Inhale deeply and raise your body upright. Repeat these steps several times.

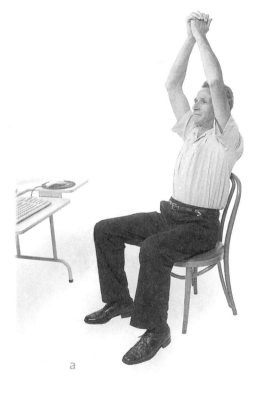

a

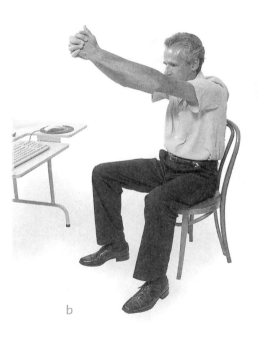

b

Benefits: The Lumberjack Pose improves your circulation, encourages deeper breathing, and is an instant energizer.

Office Tip: It is better than coffee at your desk! Replace that cup of coffee with a few repetitions of the Lumberjack Pose for an instant energy boost.

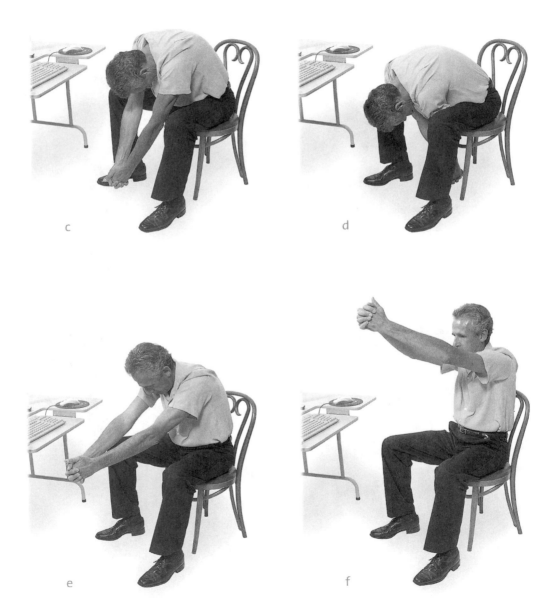

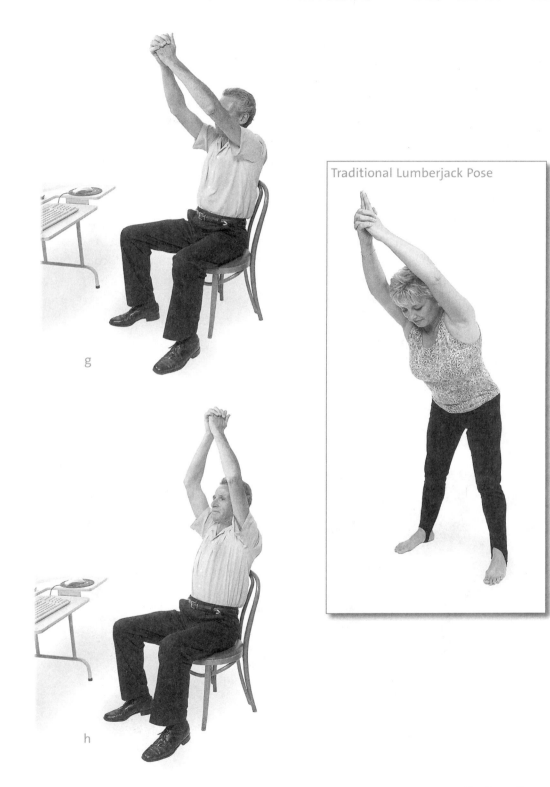

g

h

Traditional Lumberjack Pose

Yoga Mudra

Stand tall, facing the chair. Interlace your fingers behind your back. Take a deep breath and, on the exhale, squeeze your shoulder blades toward each other. If you are able, bring the heels of your hands together. Take another deep breath and, on the exhale, bend your knees slightly, press your hips and thigh creases backward, allowing your torso to bend forward. Place the crown of your head on the chair seat. Readjust the position of your hips and knees as needed. There should be very little weight on your head. Keep squeezing the shoulder blades toward each other, away from your ears, and visualize them moving toward your buttocks. Remain here for several breaths. To prevent yourself from getting light-headed, come out of the pose slowly and gently, with your chin tucked toward your chest. Come

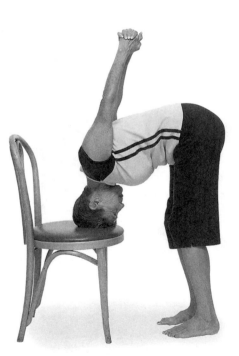

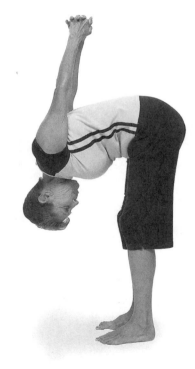

Var.

to a standing position, rounding your back, one vertebrae at a time.

Yoga Mudra can be practiced without a chair if you have good balance. If you have very tight shoulders you can use a strap, scarf, or belt as an aid.

Benefits: This pose promotes blood flow to your head. It lengthens the backs of your legs and stretches your upper back and shoulders. It aids in sinus drainage and helps alleviate allergy symptoms.

Var.

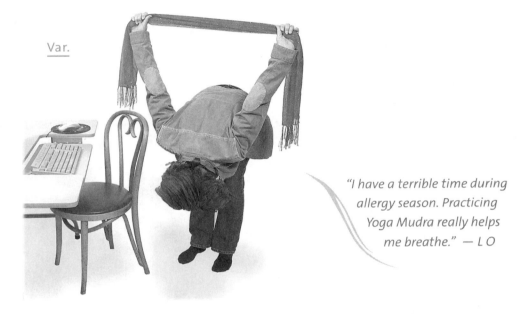

"I have a terrible time during allergy season. Practicing Yoga Mudra really helps me breathe." — L O

Traditional Yoga Mudra

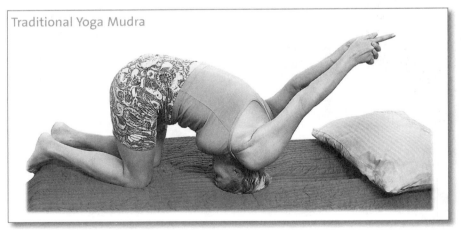

Eagle Pose

Sit comfortably toward the front of your chair. Take a few deep, conscious breaths. Stretch your arms out to your sides at shoulder level. On an exhale, bring the arms forward and cross your left elbow under your right elbow. Intertwine your arms like the fibers of a rope, with your fingers pointing to the sky. If you would like to deepen your stretch, inhale and press your arms away from your body and lift them toward the ceiling. For the lower body, cross your right ankle over the left and rest your foot or toes on the

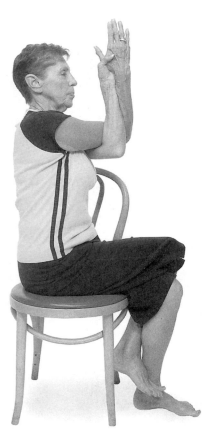

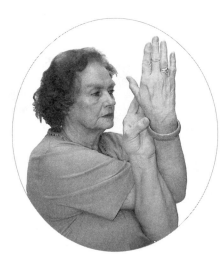

floor. If you are more flexible, wrap your right foot behind your left calf. Once you have taken several breaths, gently unfold your arms and legs and rest. Repeat the pose with your right elbow under the left, and your left leg over the right.

Benefits: This pose relieves stiffness and tension in your neck and shoulders. It opens your upper back and stretches your arms and wrists. It also stretches your feet, legs, and ankles. The squeezing action of the armpits and the thigh creases encourages lymph flow.

Tip: When traveling, try a modified Eagle Pose during the flight in the comfort of your own seat to promote lymph and blood flow.

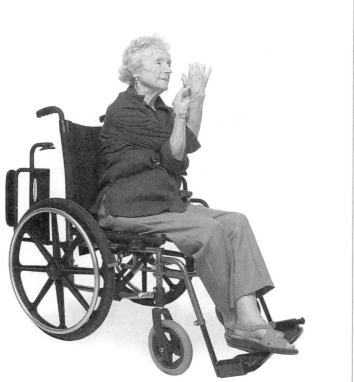

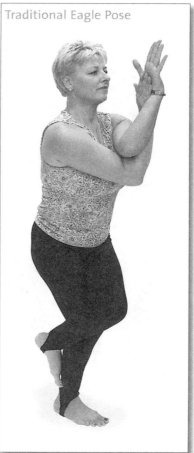

Traditional Eagle Pose

Cow-Face Pose

Sit forward in your chair. Inhale, stretch your left arm forward, bend your elbow, and reach over your left shoulder as if you were zipping up your dress. Using your right hand, gently coax your left elbow backward. Take several breaths. On an inhale, extend your right arm forward and then wrap it around your lower back. Gently spider-walk both hands toward each other. If your fingers do not meet, try using a prop, such as a tie, belt, scarf, or towel. Keep your chin parallel to the floor. Turning your head side-to-side will help to alleviate additional neck and shoulder tension. Continue

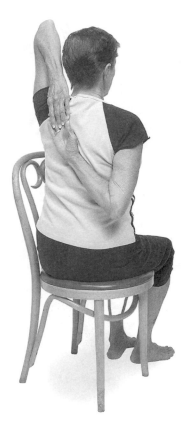

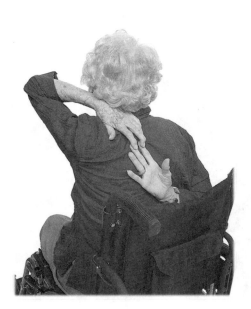

to breathe. When you feel you have had enough, release the pose. Take several breaths, noticing the differences between your right and left sides. Continue on to the opposite side, starting with the right arm.

Benefits: This pose promotes circulation in the shoulders and releases neck tension. It strengthens your upper back and pectoral muscles and opens your rib cage, allowing for deeper expansion of your lungs.

Travel Tip: While you are waiting for your flight or ride, use this pose to help relieve any tension caused by carrying luggage and shoulder bags.

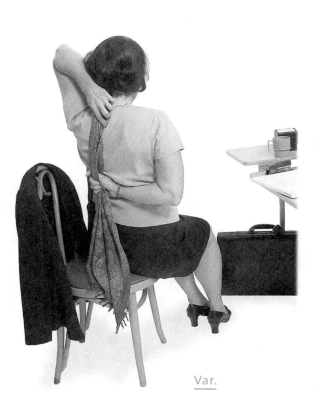

Var.

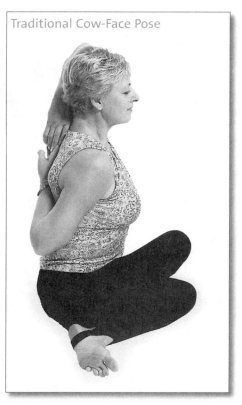

Traditional Cow-Face Pose

Fish Pose

Sitting tall toward the front edge of the chair, lean backward, resting your upper back against the chair (1). Stretch your legs out straight in front of you. On an inhale, raise both arms next to your head, drawing your relaxed shoulders away from your ears (2). Visualize a string at your breastbone, gently pulling you forward and upward, creating a comfortable arch in your back. You can look up but don't crunch the back of your neck. Be aware of the expansion of your rib cage and breathe deeply into it. Hold the pose for as long as it is comfortable for you. To release the pose, lower your hands to your sides. Holding on to the seat, slowly slide your sitting bones toward the back of the chair until you are seated upright.

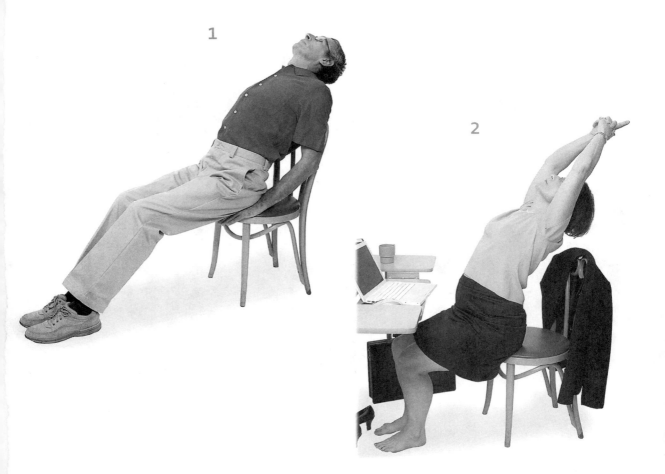

With a partner: Sit back to back. One bends forward while the other leans backward against the other partner. The one bending forward will receive a great stretch in the back of their legs and in their lower back. The one bending backward will benefit from an arch in their back that opens the chest for better respiration.

Benefits: The Fish Pose strengthens your back and releases stressed shoulders. It lengthens the front of your body and opens your rib cage for deeper breathing.

Office Tip: When you find yourself feeling fatigued at your computer, try this pose for a quick pick-me-up. It will help prevent computer hunchback and increase respiration.

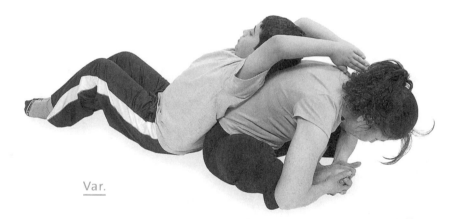

Var.

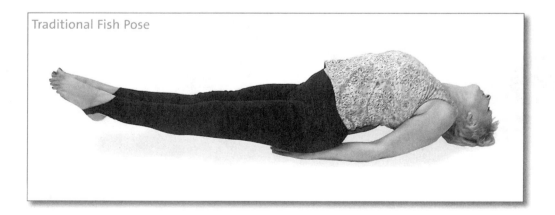

Traditional Fish Pose

Scales Pose

Sitting tall in a chair that has arms, cross your legs. If you are unable to cross your legs, leave them dangling in front of the chair or cross your ankles. With one hand on each armrest, engage your abdominal muscles and lift yourself off the chair seat. Breathe and balance here as long as you are able. When you are ready, slowly lower your buttocks to the chair, and uncross your legs. Repeat with the opposite leg crossed on top.

Benefits: Scales Pose will strengthen your wrists, hands, arms, and abdomen. It aids in relieving a compressed spine.

Travel and Office Tip: On your next flight or while in your office chair, brace your hands on the armrests. Gently raise and lower your buttocks to relieve pressure on the spinal discs.

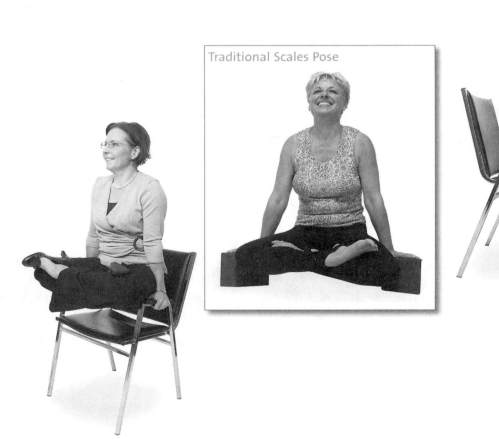

Traditional Scales Pose

Var.

Relaxation/ Meditation

Our intent when practicing yoga is to bring the mind and body together into the present moment. The following are several examples of relaxation, meditation, and visualization techniques that you can use as needed. They will help you to relax, relieve daily stress, and even fall into a deep slumber at the end of your day.

Relaxation

Seated in your chair, allow the backs
of your hands to gently rest on your
lap, with your palms facing up. Let
your shoulders relax, let your thighs
go heavy on the chair, and let your feet
go heavy on the floor.

Close your eyes. Remind yourself
to let go of any concerns from the day.
Focus on each body part and mentally
tell it to relax. As thoughts arise, put
them in a balloon and let them go.
Remain in this blissful, quiet place as

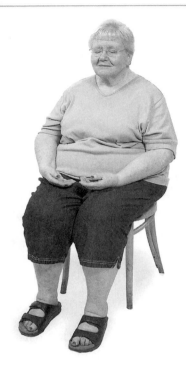

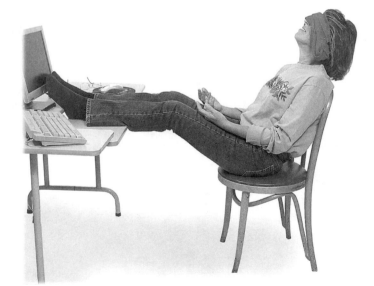

long as you like. When you are ready to move on, deepen your breath, slowly wiggle your fingers and toes and make other small movements as you wish to wake your body up. Take several deep breaths before you go about your day.

Benefits: Relaxation Pose gives you an opportunity to relax every nerve and muscle in your body. It improves respiration and focuses your energy in a positive way. It is beneficial for those suffering from heart conditions and high blood pressure.

Tip: At your desk, sit in one chair and rest your legs on another chair. On your bed, lay on your back and place your arms alongside your body with your palms facing up. Let your legs relax. If your feet want to splay out to the side, let them. Close your eyes and use an eye pillow to keep the light out. If you wish, place a small pillow under your head, neck, or knees.

Following your yoga practice, take several minutes to relax. This time aids your nervous system in integrating all of the wonderful breathing and stretching you have done.

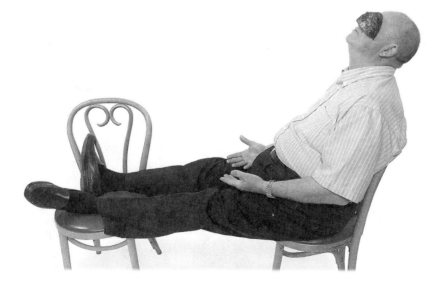

Sa-Ta-Na-Ma

Sitting tall in your chair, gently touch each finger pad to your thumb in sequence, beginning with your index finger and ending with your pinkie finger. Simultaneously, quietly or out loud, chant the syllables *Sa, Ta, Na, Ma*. Each round begins with the index finger and the syllable *Sa*. Repeat for three minutes or longer.

Benefits: This meditation activates the pressure points that help energy flow along the meridians to your brain. It aids in clearing your mind and balancing the two brain hemispheres. It stimulates the pineal and pituitary glands and calms the nervous system.

Travel Tip: Travel anxiety got you? Try this meditation while in the airport waiting to board or during takeoff.

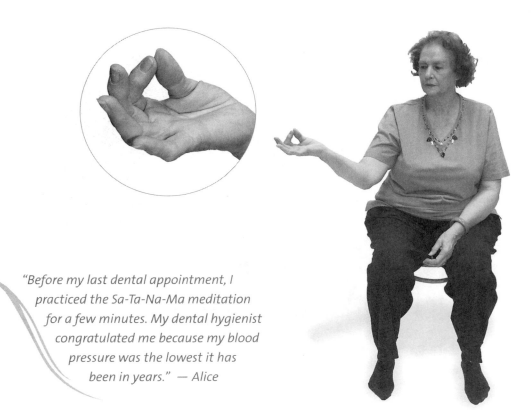

"Before my last dental appointment, I practiced the Sa-Ta-Na-Ma meditation for a few minutes. My dental hygienist congratulated me because my blood pressure was the lowest it has been in years." — Alice

Meditation for Insomnia

Lying comfortably on your bed, visualize your head becoming heavy and then allow it to sink into your pillow. Sense your neck becoming heavy, followed by your shoulders, your right arm and hand, your left arm and hand, your chest, your stomach, your hips, your right leg and foot, and then your left leg and foot. All feel heavy. If by this time you are not already sleeping, repeat the process beginning at the feet and moving upward. Pleasant dreams!

Tip: Can't sleep? Try this progressive relaxation technique slowly and with a passive mind.

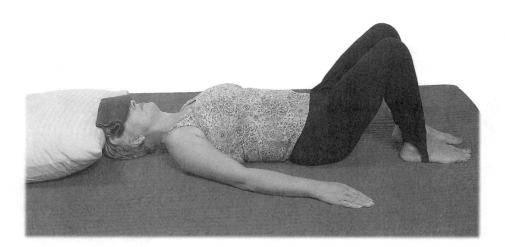

Easy-Breath Meditation

Sitting tall, take several deep-cleansing breaths. With intention, slowly raise your hands in front of your chest in Prayer Pose. Allow the knuckles of your thumbs to gently rest on your breastbone, with the finger pads of both of your hands touching each other. Consciously relax your shoulders and elbows and gently lift your breastbone. Feel your feet connecting you to the earth below and the crown of your head gently lifting upward, connecting you to the heavens above. Continue to breathe in and out through your nose. Notice the warmth or coolness of your breath as it enters your nostrils. Feel it moving down your throat as it makes its way into your lungs. With each inhale and exhale, feel the gentle rise and fall of your belly, your chest, and your rib cage. Continue this easy meditation for as long as you like.

Benefits: This meditation calms wandering thoughts. It also aids in anxiety relief and may stabilize blood pressure.

Tip: Try this meditation in a public place. It is just as effective practiced with your hands resting on your lap or thighs.

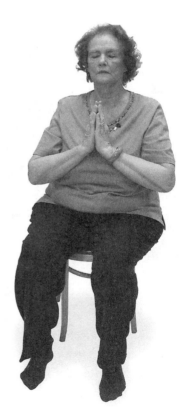

"During a recent MRI, I practiced the breath meditation that I learned in yoga and went to 'my quiet place.' It relaxed me so well that I fell asleep. I find myself going to 'my quiet place' more frequently." — *Letitia*

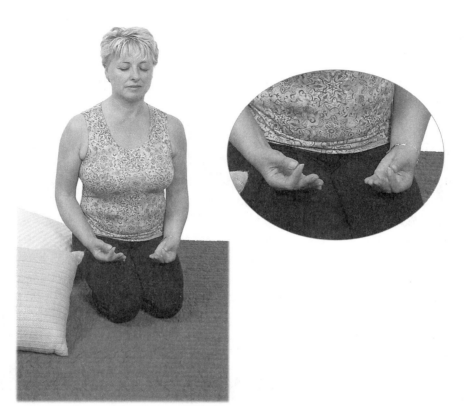

Eyes Open—Anywhere, Anytime Meditation

At the mall, the airport, or any public place: With open eyes and sitting comfortably, look down at people's feet as they walk by. Allow your breath to flow in and out through your nose as you focus on the passing feet. Allow your mind to be still. It is the movement outside of you and the quietness within you that creates stillness.

Eyes Closed—Anywhere, Anytime Meditation

With your eyes closed, tune in to the noises around you: people talking, babies crying, music blaring, the refrigerator humming, the ticking of a clock, etc.... Allow yourself to fall into the sounds until you become quiet on the inside.

Resources

Books

Anderson, Sandra, and Rolf Sovik. *Yoga: Mastering the Basics*. Honesdale, PA: Himalayan Institute Press, 2007.

Austin, Miriam. *Cool Yoga Tricks*. New York: Ballantine Books, 2003.

Bersma, Danielle, and Marjoke Visscher. *Yoga Games for Children*. Alameda, CA: Hunter House Publishers, 2003.

Christensen, Alice. *The American Yoga Association Wellness Book*. New York: Kensington Publishing, 1996.

Goldstein, Joan, and Manuela Soares. *The Joy Within: A Beginner's Guide to Meditation*. New York: Simon and Schuster, 1992.

Iyengar, B. K. S. *Light on Yoga: The Bible of Modern Yoga*. London: Thorsons, 2001.

Iyengar, B. K. S. *Yoga, The Path to Holistic Health*. New York: Dorling Kindersley Publishers Ltd, 2008.

Kabat-Zinn, John. *Wherever You Go, There You Are: Mindfulness Meditation in Everyday Life*. New York: Hyperion Books, 1994.

Maddern, Jan. *Yoga Builds Bones*. New Delhi, India: Leads Press, 2008.

McCall, Timothy. *Yoga as Medicine: The Yogic Prescription for Health & Healing*. New York, Bantam Books, 2007.

Payne, Larry, and Richard Usatine. *Yoga Rx*. New York: Broadway Books, 2002.

Purperhart, Helen. *The Yoga Adventure for Children*. Alameda, CA: Hunter House Publishers, 2007.

Purperhart, Helen. *Yoga Exercises for Teens*. Alameda, CA: Hunter House Publishers, 2009

Sanford, Matthew. *Waking*. Emmaus, PA: Rodale Books, 2008.

Scaravelli, Vanda. *Awakening the Spine*. New York: HarperOne, 1991.

Stearn, Jess. *Yoga, Youth & Reincarnation*. A. R. E. Press, 1997.

Yogananda, Paramahansa. *Autobiography of a Yogi*. Los Angeles, CA: Self-Realization Fellowship, 2006.

Websites

www.himalayaninstitute.org
  Yoga + Joyful Living

www.yogajournal.com
  Yoga Journal

www.iayt.org
  International Association of Yoga Therapists

www.lotushealingvillage.com
  Lotus Healing Village—the author's website

www.yogaalliance.org
  Yoga Alliance

www.americanyogaassociation.org
  The American Yoga Association

www.laughteryoga.org
  Laughter Yoga International